Praise for
THIS IS GOING TO HURT

"Darkly funny. . . . Heartbreaking."

—Sam Knight, *The New Yorker*

"Hilarious and heartbreaking—I howled, yelped and occasionally choked with laughter. This book may hurt, but in an important and necessary wany."

—Cathy Rentzenbrink, *The Times* (London),
"Humour Book of the Year"

"It's so hilarious. It's so irreverent, both about himself, the patients, the doctors in charge of him, that I think I laughed on every page."

—Kristan Higgins, *Entertainment Weekly*

"Blisteringly funny."

—*Boston Globe*

"So clinically funny and politically important that it should be given out on prescription."

—*The Guardian*

"At once hilarious and shocking, moving and irreverent, *This Is Going to Hurt* is a book that demands to be read."

—Maggie O'Farrell, author of *Hamnet*

"Brilliant. Five stars. Amazing."

—Mark Haddon, author of *The Curious Incident of the Dog in the Night-Time*

"A heartening, laugh-out-loud confessional on the indignities and quiet joys of being a junior doctor. Kay's warts-and-all account will not only bring plenty of laughs but also delivers a moving report from the NHS's embattled front line."

—*Financial Times*

"Scalpel-sharp humour and searing insight."

—*The Sun*

"We know that junior doctors have it rough. But it takes Kay's account of his ninety-seven-hour-week struggle to see just how rough. There are many hilariously gruesome anecdotes in this book. Some are just hilarious."

—*Sunday Times*

"The humour is unflinching in its darkness, yet I did laugh. A lot. Kay is a skillful, muscular writer, his narrative swinging from laugh-out-loud anecdotes to tales of sheer horror."

—*The Independent*

"Adam Kay writes with scalpel-sharp wit—a genital-warts-and-all account of what life is really like for junior doctors. Witty, wise and frequently moving, *This Is Going to Hurt* should be required reading for anyone who wants to be a doctor. And, frankly, anyone who might expect to cross a hospital's threshold."

—*Mail on Sunday*

"If you read one book this year, make it Adam Kay's hilarious, horrifying, heartbreaking insight into the life of a junior doctor. . . . An eye-opening and brutally funny insight into the appalling pressure upon the NHS. What a terrible loss Adam Kay is to the medical profession. But what a tremendous gain for your bookshelf."

—*Daily Express*

"Blisteringly funny, politically enraging and often heartbreaking."
—*Sunday Express*

"Painfully funny. The pain and the funniness somehow add up to something entirely good, entirely noble and entirely loveable."

—Stephen Fry

"Bloody funny."

—Minnie Driver

"Both laugh out loud funny, and incredibly sad—and only deepened my appreciation of what health care workers do."
—Jacinda Ardern, Prime Minister of New Zealand

"Adam Kay writes so beautifully, and the book is equally hilarious and devastating. . . . An extremely important read."
—*Marie Claire*

THIS IS GOING TO HURT

THIS IS GOING TO HURT

SECRET DIARIES
OF A YOUNG DOCTOR

ADAM KAY

MARINER BOOKS

Boston   New York

HarperCollins books may be purchased for educational, business, or sales promotional use. For information, please email the Special Markets Department at SPsales@harpercollins.com.

Originally published in the UK in September 2017 by Picador.

First U.S. hardcover published in December 2019 by Little, Brown Spark.

FIRST MARINER BOOKS TV TIE-IN EDITION PUBLISHED 2021.

Library of Congress Cataloging-in-Publication Data has been applied for.

ISBN 978-0-06-322848-1

22 23 24 25 26   LSC   10 9 8 7 6 5 4 3 2 1

To James,
for his wavering support

And to me,
without whom this book would
not have been possible

To respect the privacy of those friends and colleagues who might not wish to be recognized, I have altered various personal details. To maintain patient confidentiality, I have changed clinical information that might identify any individuals, altered dates,[*] and anonymized names.[†] Although fuck knows why—they can't threaten to revoke my license anymore.

---

[*] I worked a lot on labor wards, and people tend to remember the dates their kids were born.

[†] I have generally used the names of minor Harry Potter characters, to substitute one legal nightmare for another.

Contents

THIS IS GOING TO HURT

Introduction

In 2010, after six years of training and a further six years slugging it out on the hospital wards, I quit my job as a doctor. My parents still haven't forgiven me.

Sorry for the spoiler, by the way, but you knew the iceberg was coming in *Titanic*, and you watched that all the same.

When my diaries were first published in the UK, I thought I'd written a very particular, parochial book about the life of a doctor in the National Health Service. But I was—not for the first time in my life—quite extravagantly wrong. It has now been translated into thirty-seven separate languages, amounting to nearly three million copies, and I get regular e-mails from doctors in Belarus and Bogotá, in Barcelona and Bangkok, telling me, "This could have been set in my hospital." Not to mention from countless doctors in the States who've read imported or (ahem) bootlegged copies and say exactly the same. However a health-care system might be set up or funded, the experience of being a doctor is utterly universal. The same heart-break, the same hilarity, the same damaging work schedule, and, of course, the same baffling array of objects getting constantly inserted into orifices.

I should still give you a very quick primer about our health-care system; unlike an intern's first day on the wards, I won't drop you in the deep end, breeze off, and expect you to know exactly what's going on. The NHS was founded on the principle that it's free at the point of delivery and you're treated according to clinical need, not ability to pay—whether you live in Windsor Castle or on a bench outside Windsor Station. Other systems around the world might be more efficient, but I'd drag myself out of a coma to argue that none of them is fairer.

Universal health care is obviously a bit of a political hot potato on your side of the pond, but—much like ant-egg soup or a night of bukkake—don't knock it till you've tried it. Here in the UK, you don't have to check your bank-account balance after booking an appointment or delay treatment until your finances allow it, and (ahem, again) no one ever faces bankruptcy because of medical bills.

Like the health system's other 1.4 million employees, I will always feel tremendously proud to say I worked for the NHS. It's unlike any other national asset; no one speaks fondly about the Bank of England or the London Underground. The NHS fixed our broken arms on field day, gave our grandmas chemotherapy, treated the chlamydia we brought back from spring break, started us on inhalers—and all this wizardry was free and right when we needed it.

So you'll forgive me for feeling sentimental when, a few years ago, the GMC (General Medical Council— the bastards who regulate doctors in the UK) wrote to say they were taking my name off the medical register. It wasn't a massive shock, as I hadn't practiced medicine in half a decade, but it was still a huge emotional wrench to permanently close that chapter of my life.

It was, however, excellent news for my spare room, as I cleared out box upon box of old paperwork, shredding files faster than Willie Nelson's accountant. I couldn't quite let all of it go, rescuing from the jaws of death my training portfolio, where doctors log their clinical experiences. On flicking through its curling pages for the first time in years, I remembered shuffling up to my hospital on-call room between crises and scrawling down anything remotely interesting that had happened that day like a blood-spattered, epically tired Samuel Pepys.

Reading back over it, I was reminded of the brutal hours and the colossal impact being a junior doctor had on my life. It now seemed extreme and unreasonable in terms of what was expected of me, but at the time, I'd just accepted it as part of the job. The extra mile was the normal distance. I wouldn't have flinched if an entry read *swam to Iceland for prenatal clinic* or *had to eat a helicopter today*. I truly believe that anyone who ever has or ever will encounter a doctor should better understand what it's like to be on the other side of the scalpel, should get to peek behind the scrubs, the gloves, and the calm demeanor. So here they are, the diaries I kept during my time as a doctor, genital warts and all. What it was really like on the front line, how my personal life became a hobby I never had time for, and how, one terrible day, it all became too much for me and I finally hit the iceberg.

Come on in, the water's lovely.

1

House Officer

The decision to work in medicine is basically a version of the e-mail you get in early October asking you to choose your menu options for the work Christmas party. No doubt you'll choose the chicken, to be on the safe side, and it's more than likely everything will be all right. But what if someone shares a ghastly factory-farming video on Facebook the day before and you inadvertently witness a mass debeaking and then turn your back on a lifestyle thus far devoted almost exclusively to consuming meat? What if you develop a life-threatening allergy to scallops? Ultimately, there's no way to know what you'll fancy for dinner in sixty dinners' time.

In the UK, would-be doctors make their career choices at age sixteen, two years before they're legally allowed to text a photo of their own genitals. When you sit down and tick *medicine* on an application form, you're set off on a trajectory that continues until you either retire or die, and, unlike your work Christmas party, Janet from procurement won't swap your chicken for her halloumi skewers—you're stuck with it.

Whatever my misgivings about the costs of the American health-care system, I have no doubt in my mind that something you've got absolutely right is sticking medical school after a bachelor's; getting a medical degree is a decision you should make in your early twenties, not as a teenager. When you're sixteen, your reasons for wanting to pursue a career in medicine are generally along the lines of "My mum/dad's a doctor," "I quite like *Grey's Anatomy*," or "I want to cure cancer." Reasons one and two are ludicrous, and reason three would be perfectly fine—if a little earnest—were it not for the fact that that's what research scientists do, not doctors. Besides, holding anyone to his word at that age seems a bit unfair, on par with declaring the "I want to be an astronaut" painting you did at age five a legally binding document.

Personally, I don't remember medicine ever being an active career decision; it was more just the default setting for my life—the marimba ringtone, the stock photo of a mountain range as your computer background. I grew up in a Jewish family (although they were mostly in it for the food); went to the kind of school that's essentially a sausage factory designed to churn out doctors, lawyers, and politicians; and my dad was a doctor. It was written on the wall.

Because medical schools have ten times more applicants than positions available, all candidates must be interviewed, and only those who perform best under a grilling are awarded a place. It's assumed all applicants will receive top marks in their exams, so universities base their selections on nonacademic criteria. This, of course, makes sense; doctors must be psychologically fit for the job—able to make decisions under a terrifying amount of pressure, able to break bad news to anguished relatives, able to deal with death on a daily basis. They must have something that cannot be memorized and graded; a great doctor must have a huge heart and a distended aorta through which pumps a vast lake of compassion and human kindness.

At least, that's what you'd think. In reality, medical schools don't give the shiniest shit about any of that. They don't even check if you're okay with the sight of blood. Instead, they fixate on extracurricular activities. Their ideal student is captain of two sports teams, the county swimming champion, leader of the youth orchestra, and editor of the school newspaper. It's basically a Miss Congeniality contest without the sash. Look at the Wikipedia entry for any famous doctor, and you'll see something along the lines of "He was an accomplished rugby player in youth leagues. He excelled as a distance runner and in his final year at school served as vice-captain of the athletics team." This particular description is of Harold Shipman—a family doctor who murdered over two hundred of his patients—so perhaps it's not a totally rock-solid system.

The University of London seemed satisfied that my distinctions in grade eight piano and saxophone, alongside some half-arsed theater reviews for the school magazine, qualified me perfectly for life on the wards, so in 1998 I packed my bags and embarked upon the treacherous six-mile journey from my suburb in southeast London to university.

As you might imagine, learning every single aspect of the human body's anatomy and physiology plus each possible way it can malfunction is a fairly gargantuan undertaking. But the buzz of knowing I was going to become a doctor one day—such a big deal, you get to literally change your name, like a superhero or an international criminal—propelled me toward my goal through those long years.

Then there I was, a junior doctor. *Junior doctor* is the term we use to describe any hospital doctor who isn't a consultant (or, as you'd have it, an attending physician). Junior doctors are divided into the ranks of house officer, senior house officer, registrar, and senior registrar. Got it? Oh. Okay, how about if I draw you a chart?

US terminology	UK terminology
Intern	House officer (junior doctor)
Resident	Senior house officer (SHO) (junior doctor)
Fellow	Registrar (junior doctor)
	Senior registrar (junior doctor)
Attending physician	Consultant (senior doctor)

Now it was finally time to step out onto the ward armed with all my exhaustive knowledge and turn theory into practice. My spring couldn't have been coiled any tighter. So it came as quite the blow to discover that I'd spent a quarter of my life at medical school and it hadn't remotely prepared me for the Jekyll-and-Hyde existence of a house officer.

During the day, the job was manageable, if mind-numbing and insanely time-consuming. You turn up every morning for ward rounds, where your whole team of doctors rambles past each of their patients. You trail behind like a hypnotized duckling, your head cocked to one side in a caring manner, noting down every pronouncement from your seniors—book an MRI, refer to rheumatology, arrange an ECG. Then you spend the rest of your working day (plus generally a further unpaid four hours) completing these dozens, sometimes hundreds, of tasks—filling in forms, making phone calls. Essentially, you're a glorified personal assistant. Not really what I'd trained so hard for, but whatever.

The night shifts, however, made Dante look like Disney—an unrelenting nightmare that made me regret ever thinking my education was being underutilized. At night, the house officer is given a little paging device affectionately called a bleeper and responsibility for every patient in the hospital. The fucking lot of them. The nighttime SHO and registrar will be down in the ER seeing and admitting patients while you're up on the wards, sailing the ship alone. A ship that's enormous, and on fire, and that no one has really taught you how to sail. You've been trained on how to examine a patient's cardiovascular system, you know the physiology of the coronary vasculature, but recognizing every sign and symptom of a heart attack is very different than actually managing one.

You're bleeped by ward after ward, nurse after nurse, with emergency after emergency—it never stops, all night long. Your senior colleagues are seeing patients in the ER with specific problems, like pneumonia or broken legs. Your patients are having similar emergencies, but they're hospital inpatients, meaning they already had something significantly wrong with them in the first place. It's a "build your own burger" of symptoms layered on conditions layered on diseases; you see a patient with pneumonia who was admitted with liver failure or a patient who's broken her leg falling out of bed after another epileptic fit. You're a one-man, mobile, essentially untrained ER, getting drenched in bodily fluids (not even the fun kind), seeing an endless stream of worryingly sick patients who, twelve hours earlier, had an entire team of doctors caring for them. You suddenly long for the sixteen-hour admin sessions. (Or, ideally, some kind of compromise job that's neither massively beyond nor beneath your abilities.)

It's sink or swim, and you have to learn how to swim because otherwise a ton of patients sink with you. I actually found it all perversely exhilarating. Sure, it was hard work; sure, the hours were bordering on inhuman; and sure, I saw things that have scarred my retinas to this day, but I was a doctor now.

Tuesday, August 3, 2004

Day one. H* has made me a packed lunch. I have a new stethoscope,† a new shirt, and a new e-mail address: atom.kay@nhs.net. It's good to know that no matter what happens today, nobody can accuse me of being the most incompetent person in the hospital. And even if I am, I can blame it on Atom.

I'm enjoying the ice-breaking potential of the story, but in the pub afterward, my anecdote is rather trumped by my friend Amanda's. Amanda's surname is Saunders-Vest. They have spelled out the hyphen in her name, making her amanda.saundershyphenvest@nhs.net.

Wednesday, August 18, 2004

Patient OM is a seventy-year-old retired heating engineer from Manchester, but tonight he will be play-

---

* H was my short-suffering partner. Don't worry, you're not going to have to remember huge numbers of characters. It's not *Game of Thrones.*

† I'm all for explaining terminology as we go along, but if you don't know what a stethoscope is, this is probably a book to regift.

ing the role of an eccentric German professor with ze unconvinzing agzent. Not just tonight, in fact, but this morning, this afternoon, and every day of his admission thanks to his dementia, exacerbated by a urinary tract infection.[*]

Professor OM's favorite routine is to follow behind the doctors on ward rounds, his hospital gown on back to front, like a white coat (plus or minus underwear, for a bit of morning bratwurst), and chime in with "Yes," "Zat is correct," and the occasional "Genius!" whenever a doctor says something.

On consultant and registrar ward rounds, I escort him back to his bed immediately and make sure the nursing staff keep him tucked in for a couple of hours. On my solo rounds, I let him tag along for a bit. I don't particularly know what I'm doing, and I don't have vast depths of confidence even when I do, so it's actually quite helpful to have a superannuated German cheerleader behind me shouting out "Zat is brilliant!" every so often.

Today he took a dump on the floor next to me, so, sadly, I had to retire him from active duty.

---

[*]   Urinary tract infections, or any kind of low-grade sepsis, often make the elderly go a bit nuts.

Monday, August 30, 2004

Whatever we lack in free time, we more than make up for in stories about patients. Today in the mess* over lunch we're trading stories about nonsense symptoms that people have presented with. Between us in the last few weeks, we've seen patients with itchy teeth, sudden *improvement* in hearing, and arm pain during urination. Each one gets a polite ripple of laughter, like a local dignitary's speech at a graduation ceremony. We go round the table sharing our version of campfire ghost stories until it's Seamus's turn. He tells us he saw someone in the ER this morning who thought he was sweating on only half his face.

He sits back in anticipation of bringing the house down, but there's merely silence. Until pretty much everyone chimes in with "So, Horner's syndrome, then?" He's never heard of it, specifically not the fact that it likely indicates a lung tumor. Seamus scrapes his chair back with an earsplitting screech and dashes off to make a phone call to get the patient back to the department. I finish his Twix.

---

* The *doctors' mess* refers to either our communal area with a few sofas and a dilapidated pool table or the state of most of my patients in the first few months.

Friday, September 10, 2004

I notice that every patient on the ward has a pulse of 60 recorded in the observation chart so I surreptitiously inspect the health-care assistant's measurement technique. He feels the patient's pulse, looks at his watch, and meticulously counts the number of seconds per minute.

Sunday, October 17, 2004

To give myself a bit of credit, I didn't panic when the patient I was seeing on the ward unexpectedly started hosing enormous quantities of blood out of his mouth and onto my shirt. To give myself no credit whatsoever, I didn't know what else to do. I asked the nearest nurse to get Hugo, my registrar, who was on the next ward, and meantime I put in a Venflo* and ran some fluids. Hugo arrived before I could do anything else, which was handy, as I was completely out of ideas by

---

* A *Venflon*, or *cannula*, is the plastic tube that gets shoved into a vessel in the back of the hand or the crook of an elbow so we can run drugs or fluids intravenously through a drip. Putting in Venflons is one of the key responsibilities of a house officer, although I got through medical school without ever having tried it. On the night before my first day as a doctor, one of my flatmates in our on-site hospital accommodation stole a box of about eighty of them from a ward and we practiced cannulating ourselves for a few hours until we could finally do it. We were covered in track marks for days.

that point. Start looking for the patient's stopcock? Shove loads of paper towels down his throat? Float some basil in it and declare it gazpacho?

Hugo diagnosed esophageal varices,* which made sense, as the patient was the color of Homer Simpson— from the early series, when the contrast was much more extreme and everyone looked like a cave painting—and he tried to control the bleeding with a Sengstaken tube.† As the patient flailed around, resisting this awful thing going down his throat, the blood jetted everywhere—on me, on Hugo, on the walls, curtains, ceiling. It was like a particularly avant-garde episode of *Fixer Upper*. The sound was the worst part. With every breath the poor man took, you could hear the blood being sucked down into his lungs, choking him.

By the time the tube was inserted, he'd stopped bleeding. Bleeding always stops eventually, and this was for the saddest reason. Hugo pronounced the patient dead, wrote up the notes, and asked the nurse to inform the family. I peeled off my bloodsoaked clothes and we silently changed into scrubs. So there we go, the first death I've ever witnessed and every bit as horrific as it could possibly have been. Nothing romantic or beautiful about it. That sound. Hugo took me out-

---

* *Varices* are a horrible complication of liver cirrhosis where you essentially get huge varicose veins inside your esophagus that can rupture at any point and bleed heavily.

† A tube you can wedge down the throat that—when it's in position—can be inflated like a balloon to put pressure on the vessels and hopefully stop the bleeding.

side for a cigarette—we both desperately needed one after that. And I'd never smoked before.

Tuesday, November 9, 2004

Bleeped awake at three a.m. from my first half-hour's shuteye in three shifts to go to the ward and prescribe a sleeping pill for a patient, whose sleep is evidently much more important than mine. My powers are greater than I realized—I arrive on the ward to find the patient is asleep.

Friday, November 12, 2004

An inpatient's lab results show her clotting process is all over the map for no good reason. Hugo eventually cracks it. She has been taking St. John's wort capsules from a health-food store for anxiety. Hugo points out to her (and, in fairness, me) that it interacts with the metabolism of her warfarin, and her clotting will probably settle down if she stops taking it. She is astonished. "I thought it was just herbal—how can it be that bad for you?"

As soon as she says the words *just herbal*, the temperature in the room seems to drop a few degrees and Hugo barely holds in a weary sigh. It's clearly not his first time at this particular rodeo.

"Apricot stones contain cyanide," he replies drily.

"The death cap mushroom has a fifty percent fatality rate. *Natural* does not equal *safe*. There's a plant in my garden that if you simply sat under it for ten minutes, you'd be dead." Job done; she tosses the tablets.

I ask him about that plant over a colonoscopy later. "Water lily."

Monday, December 6, 2004

All junior doctors at the hospital have been asked to sign a document opting out of the European Working Time Directive* because our contracts are noncompliant with it. This week I have seen H for under two hours and worked for a grand total of ninety-seven. *Noncompliant* doesn't quite seem to cover it. My contract has taken the directive, dragged it screaming from its bed in the dead of night, and waterboarded it.

Thursday, January 20, 2005

Dear drug-dealing bastard,

Over the last few nights, we've had to admit three young patients, all dry as a husk, basically

---

* The European Working Time Directive was brought in to provide some legal measure to stop employers working their staff to their bleary-eyed deaths by limiting shifts to a "mere" forty-eight hours per week.

collapsed through hypotension, and with their electrolytes fucked up.[*]

The only connection among these individuals is their recent use of cocaine. For all its heart-attacking, septum-shrinking risks, cocaine does not cause this to happen to people. What I'm pretty confident is going on here—and I want a Nobel Prize at the very least if I'm right—is that you've been bulking out your supply with your nan's furosemide.[†]

Aside from the fact that you're wasting my evenings and my unit's beds, it feels like fairly terrible business practice to be hospitalizing your customers. Kindly use chalk like everyone else.

Yours faithfully,
Dr. Adam Kay

---

[*] *Electrolytes* are the salts in the blood, mostly sodium, potassium, chloride, and calcium. If levels become too high or too low, your body alerts you by making your heart stop or putting you in a coma. It's clever like that.

[†] Furosemide is a diuretic; if you've got a buildup of fluid in your lungs or tissues, generally from a malfunctioning heart or kidneys, it will make you pee it out. If you don't have a buildup of fluid, as here, it will make you pee out the water content of your blood.

Monday, January 31, 2005

Saved a life tonight. I was bleeped to see a sixty-eight-year-old inpatient who was as close to death's door as it's possible to be—he'd already pressed the bell and was peering through the frosted glass into the Grim Reaper's hallway. His oxygen saturation[*] was 73 percent—I suspect if the vending machine hadn't been out of order and I'd bought my Snickers as planned, it would have all been too late.

I didn't even have the spare seconds to run through the bullet points of a management plan in my head—I just started performing action after action on an autopilot mode I didn't know I possessed. Oxygen on, intravenous access, blood tests, blood gases, diuretics, catheter. He started to perk up pretty much immediately, the bungee rope jerking him back from a millimeter above the concrete. Sorry, Death—you're one short for your dinner party this evening. By the time Hugo arrived, I felt like Superman.

A strange realization that it's the first time I've actually saved a life in five months as a doctor. Everyone on the outside imagines we roam the wards performing routine acts of heroism; I even assumed that myself when I started. The truth is, although dozens, maybe hundreds, of lives are saved every day on hospital

---

[*] *Oxygen saturation* is the percentage of oxygen in your blood, and it's measured by that little clip they put on the end of your finger. It should be as close to 100 percent as possible, definitely above 90 percent, and *definitely* definitely above 80 percent.

wards, almost every time it happens, it's in a much more low-key, team-based way. It's not a doctor performing a single action so much as him implementing a sensible plan that gets carried out by any number of colleagues who at every stage check to see if the patient is getting better and modify the plan if he's not.

But sometimes it *is* down to one person, and today, for the first time, it was me. Hugo seems happy, or at least as happy as he's capable of being: "Well, you've bought him another couple of weeks on earth." Come on—give a superhero a break here.

Monday, February 7, 2005

My move to surgery* has rewarded me with my very first degloving injury.†

Patient WM is eighteen and was out celebrating with friends. After closing time he found himself dancing on the roof of a bus shelter, then decided to descend to ground level using a handy neighboring lamppost as a fireman's pole. He jumped over to the lamppost and slid down, koala-bear-style. He unfortunately

---

* House officers generally spend six months working in medicine and six months in surgery. The very shortest of straws saw me working in urology, a surgical subspecialty.

† A *degloving injury* is where skin is traumatically torn from the underlying tissues; it's typically seen in motorcycle accidents, where the rider's hands drag along the ground. Rats are able to deglove their tails at will to escape capture. Quite why we were taught this in medical school escapes me.

misjudged the texture of the lamppost—it wasn't the smooth ride he was expecting at all but a chafing, agonizing, gritty slump to the bottom. He therefore presented to the ER with severe grazing to both palms and a complete degloving of his penis.

I have seen a lot of penises in my brief time in urology (and beyond) but this was far and away the worst one I have ever seen. Worthy of a rosette, if only there'd been a place to pin it. A couple of inches of urethra, coated with a thin layer of bloody pulp, maybe half a centimeter diameter in total. It brought to mind a remnant of spaghetti stuck to the bottom of the bowl by a smear of tomato sauce. Perhaps not surprisingly, WM was upset. His distress was only made worse when he asked if the penis could be "regloved" and Dr. Binns, the consultant, calmly explained that the "glove" was spread evenly up eight feet of lamppost in west London.

Monday, February 21, 2005

Discharging a patient home after laparoscopy,* I sign her off work for two weeks. She offers me a tenner to

---

* Almost any abdominal operation can now be performed laparoscopically, which is Greek for "much slower" and involves inserting tiny cameras and instruments on long sticks through little holes. It's fiddly and takes a long time to learn. Re-create the experience for yourself by tying your shoelaces with chopsticks. With your eyes closed. In space.

sign her off for a month. I laugh, but she's serious and ups her offer to fifteen quid. I suggest she see her GP if she's not feeling up to work after a fortnight.

I clearly need to dress smarter if that's the level of bribe I'm attracting. On the way home I wonder how much she'd have needed to offer before I said yes. Depressingly, I put it somewhere around fifty pounds.

Monday, March 14, 2005

Out for dinner with H and some mates—a pizza restaurant with exposed brickwork, too much neon, menus on clipboards, an unnecessarily complicated ordering system, and the almost total absence of waiting staff. You're given a device that beeps and vibrates when your order is ready, whereupon you schlep across the artfully mismatched tiles to collect your pizza from an uninterested server who sits there safe in the knowledge that no one ever asks for the 12.5 percent service charge to be taken off the bill—even when no actual serving is done.

The device goes off. I say, "Oh my God," and reflexively jump to my feet. It's not that I'm particularly excited about my Fiorentina; it's just that the fucking thing has the exact same pitch and timbre as my hospital bleeper. H takes my pulse—it's 95. Work has pretty much given me PTSD.

Sunday, March 20, 2005

There's more to breaking bad news than "I'm afraid it's cancer" and "We did everything we could." Nothing can prepare you for sitting a patient's daughter down to explain that something rather upsetting happened to her frail, elderly father overnight.

I had to tell her that the patient in the bed next to her dad's became extremely agitated and confused last night. That he thought her father was in fact his own wife. That unfortunately by the time the nurses heard the commotion and attended, it was too late, and this patient was straddling her father and had ejaculated onto his face.

"At least it didn't . . . go any further than that," said the daughter in a world-class demonstration of finding the positive in a situation.

Monday, April 11, 2005

About to take a ten-year-old straight from the ER to the operating theater for a ruptured appendix. Colin, a charming registrar, has been conducting a master class in dealing with a worried mum—explaining everything that's going on in her son's tummy, what we're going to do to fix it, how long it'll take, when he'll be allowed to go home. I try to absorb his method. It's about telling her just the right amount—keeping her informed but not overwhelmed—and delivering everything at the right level; not too much jargon but never patronizing. Above all, it's about being professional and kind.

Her expression becomes less uneasy by the second and I can feel the angst leave her body like an evil spirit or trapped wind. It's time to take the kid upstairs, so Colin nods to the mum and says, "Quick kiss before he goes off to theater?" She leans over and pecks Colin on the cheek. Her pride and joy is wheeled away, his own cheek sadly dry.

Tuesday, May 31, 2005

Three nights ago, I admitted patient MJ, a homeless guy in his fifties, with acute pancreatitis. This was the third time we'd admitted him with acute pancreatitis since I started this job. We got him comfortable with pain relief and started him on IV fluids—he was sore and miserable.

"At least you get a warm bed for a few nights," I said. "Are you joking?" he replied. "I'll get bloody MRSA in here." It's come to something when the streets outside a hospital have a better reputation for cleanliness than the corridors within.

I don't like to preach, but I'm a doctor and not wanting him to die is kind of in the job description, so I reminded him he's in here because of alcohol,* and

---

* Pancreatitis is extremely painful, often very severe, and generally

even if I can't persuade him to stop drinking (I can't), if he could at least stay off it until we've gotten him out of the hospital, it would really help. This time, it'd be a real bonus if he wouldn't mind laying off the alcogel dispensers.

He reared back like I'd just accused him of twincest, telling me that of course he would *never* do that—they've changed the recipe recently and now it tastes really bitter. He pulled me closer to whisper in my ear that in this hospital you're best off sucking on some of the sanitizing wipes, then gave me a conspiratorial tap on the arm as if to say, *That one's on me.* Tonight he discharged himself "home," but he'll doubtless be back with us in the coming weeks.

As per tradition, my SHO and I celebrate the end of our run of night shifts and go for a slap-up breakfast and a bottle of white wine at Vingt-Quatre. Night shifts are essentially a different time zone to the rest of the country, so even though it's nine a.m., you can hardly call it an eye-opener—it's practically a nightcap. As I'm refilling our glasses, there's a knock on the window. It's MJ, who laughs uproariously before shooting me his best *I knew it!* look. I resolve to sit farther from the window next time. Or just have a quick suck on an alcohol wipe in the changing rooms.

---

caused by either alcohol or gallstones. There are a number of other causes, and the mnemonic for remembering them, pleasingly, is GET SMASHED. (The second *S* stands for "scorpion venom.")

Sunday, June 5, 2005

It would be unfair to label every single orthopedic surgeon as a bone-crunching Neanderthal simply on the basis of the 99 percent of them it applies to, but my heart does seem to sink with every nighttime bleep to their ward.

So far this weekend I've seen two of their patients. Yesterday: a man in atrial fibrillation[*] following surgery for a #NOF.[†] I note from his admission ECG he was in AF at that point too—a fact completely unnoticed by his admitting team, even though it would almost certainly explain why he ended up sprawled across the floor in a supermarket in the first place. I feel like running a teaching session for the orthopedic department entitled "Sometimes People Fall Over for a Reason."

Today, I'm asked to see a twenty-year-old patient whose blood tests show abnormal renal function. Both his arms are in full plaster casts like a *Scooby-Doo* villain's. He's got no drip for fluids and an untouched glass of water on his bedside table that—despite all the will in the world, I'm sure—physics has prevented him from touching for the past couple of days. I prescribe IV fluids for the patient, though it would be more ef-

---

[*] *Atrial fibrillation (AF)* means the heart is beating fast, erratically, and inefficiently—this isn't ideal.

[†] The notation *#NOF* means "fractured neck of femur." If you thought # was a hashtag, you're banned from reading the rest of the book.

ficient to prescribe common sense for some of my colleagues.

Tuesday, June 7, 2005

Assisting in operating theaters on the emergency list, removing a foreign object from a patient's rectum. I've been a doctor less than a year, and this is the fourth object I have removed from a rectum—professionally, at least.

My first encounter was a handsome young Italian man who arrived at the hospital with the majority of a toilet brush inside of him (bristles first) and went home with a colostomy bag. His big Italian mother was grateful in ways that Brits never are, lavishing thanks and praise on every member of staff she met for saving her son's life. She put her arm round the equally handsome young man who'd accompanied her son to the hospital. "And thank God his friend Philip was staying in the spare room at the time to call the ambulance!"

Most of these patients suffer from Eiffel syndrome— "I fell, Doctor! I fell!"—and the tales of how things get where can be skyscraper-tall (come to think of it, it's only a matter of time before someone tries to sit on the Empire State Building), but today I'd actually believed a patient's story. It was a credible and painful-sounding incident with a sofa and a remote control that at the very least had me furrowing my brow and thinking, *Well, I suppose it* could *happen*. Upon removal of the remote control in the OR, however, we noticed it had a condom on it, so maybe it wasn't a complete accident.

Thursday, June 16, 2005

I told a patient that his MRI wouldn't be until next week and he threatened to break both my legs. My first thought was *Well, it'll be a couple of weeks off work*. I was *this* close to offering to find him a baseball bat.

Saturday, June 25, 2005

Called to pronounce death* on an elderly patient—he'd been extremely sick, was DNR, and this wasn't unexpected. The staff nurse takes me to the cubicle, points out the slate-gray former patient, and introduces me to the wife, who you could say isn't technically a widow until I make the call that he's officially dead. Nature may do all the heavy lifting, but you still need me on hand to sign the form.

I extend condolences to the patient's wife and suggest she might want to wait outside while I perform

---

* Doctors are legally obliged to fill out death certificates for their patients detailing causes of death. In hospital settings, they will generally also be asked to formally pronounce (confirm) death.

some formalities, but she says she'd rather stay. I'm not sure why; I don't think she knows why either. Perhaps every moment with him matters, even if he's no longer with us, or maybe she wants to check that I'm not one of those doctors she's read about in the tabloids who do unspeakable things to the deceased. Anyway, she's settling down in her front-row seat whether I like it or not.

I've pronounced three deaths before, but this is the first time I've had a captive audience. I feel I should have laid on refreshments. She clearly doesn't realize quite how tense, silent, and drawn-out this evening's performance is going to be—more Pinter than *Priscilla, Queen of the Desert*.

I confirm the patient's identity from his hospital wristband, check visually for respiratory effort, check there's no response to verbal or physical stimuli. Feel for a carotid pulse, check with a torch that pupils are fixed and dilated. Check watch and listen with stethoscope for heart sounds for two minutes. Then listen for lung sounds for another three minutes. *Overkill* feels like an inappropriate word, but five minutes is an extraordinarily long time when you're standing motionless under brilliant white light, your stethoscope pressed against a definitely dead man's chest, observed by his grieving wife. This is why we try and get them out of the room for this bit.*

---

* When a pope dies, zero chances are taken. According to the Vatican's rules, clearly drawn up by someone who thought *The Exorcist* was on the tame side, the doctor has to call out the

The almost-widow keeps asking if I am okay. I don't know whether she thinks I'm too upset to move or have just forgotten what to do next in the death-pronouncing, but every time she says something, I leap up like . . . well, like a doctor hearing a noise while listening carefully to the chest of a corpse.

Once I peel myself off the ceiling and calm down, I confirm the sad news to her and document my findings. It was certainly an agonizing five minutes, but if the whole medicine thing goes tits-up, I'm only a tin of silver paint and an old crate away from a gig in Times Square as a living statue.

Tuesday, July 5, 2005

Trying to work out a seventy-year-old lady's alcohol consumption to record in the notes. I've established that wine is her poison.

Me: And how much wine do you drink per day, would you say?

Patient: About three bottles on a good day.

Me: Okay . . . and on a bad day?

Patient: On a bad day I only manage one.

---

pope's name three times, check the body's breath doesn't blow out a candle, then, just to be certain, bop him on the head with a hammer. At least she didn't have to watch me do that.

Thursday, July 7, 2005

Terrorist atrocities across London, major incident declared, all doctors told to report to the ER.

My responsibility was to go around the surgical wards and discharge any patient whose life or limb wasn't in immediate danger to clear the decks for new arrivals from the bombings. I was like a snowplow with a stethoscope, booting out anyone who got to the third syllable of *malingerer* without passing out or coughing up blood. Got rid of hundreds of the bed-blocking fuckers.

Wednesday, July 13, 2005

The hospital didn't receive any casualties, and with no patients I've basically done no work for a week.

Saturday, July 23, 2005

This weekend is my best mate Ron's bachelor party, and I've had to bail out with barely four hours' notice. It's annoying for a million reasons, from the fact it was just a close selection of pals with only eight of us making the cut, to the personalized T-shirts, to the now-uneven paintballing teams, to the four hundred fucking pounds I spent on it.

I was originally due to be working but arranged a

four-way swap (A doing my shift, B doing A's shift, C doing B's shift and me doing C's shift), so it was always slightly precarious, like a house purchase in a massive chain. And now C (who I've barely met before) has real or imaginary childcare issues for one of her real or imaginary children, so I'm here on the ward instead of skydiving, off my tits on tequila.

Nondoctors* struggle to understand why it doesn't actually help having loads of notice for this kind of thing; more than two months' notice means we don't have the schedule yet. I order a bottle of whiskey I can't afford—I can virtually hear Elton John saying, *Steady on, let's not go crazy here*—and arrange to have it delivered to Ron's flat on his return, along with my groveling apologies. We arrange a bachelor-party postscript for just the two of us in a fortnight's time, after my run of nights and after the three locum shifts I booked to cover the cost of the weekend I'm now missing.

Friday, July 29, 2005

I spend the entire night shift feeling like water is gushing into the hull of my boat and the only thing on hand to bail it out with is a Calico Critter's contact lens.

Everything I'm bleeped about takes at least fifteen

---

* There should be a term for nondoctors, the medical equivalent of *layperson* or *civilian*. *Patients*, maybe?

minutes to firefight, and I'm getting called about a new blaze every five minutes, so the sums don't *quite* add up. My SHO and registrar are tied up in a busy ER, so I prioritize the sickest-sounding patients and manage the expectations of the nurses who call me about anything else.

"I'm really sorry but I've got a load of patients who are much more urgent," I say. "Realistically, it'll be about six hours." Some understand and some react like I've just said, *Fuck off, I'm in the middle of an* Ally McBeal *box-set binge.* I run from chest pain to sepsis to atrial fibrillation to acute asthma all night like some kind of medical decathlon, and somehow everyone gets through it alive.

At eight a.m. one of the night nurses bleeps to tell me I did really well and she thinks I'm a good little doctor. I'm willing to overlook the fact that "good little doctor" sounds like a Nancy Drew character, because I'm pretty sure it's the first time I've had anything approaching a compliment since I got my medical license. I don't really know what to say but stutter my thanks. In my confusion, I accidentally sign off with "Love you, bye." It's partly exhaustion, partly my brain misfiring because H is normally the only person who says nice things to me, and partly because, in that moment, I genuinely loved her for saying that.

2

Senior House Officer—Post One

By August 2005, I was a senior house officer—or first-year resident, if you've forgotten the table that it took me nearly an hour to work out how to draw on Microsoft Word. I was obviously still extremely junior, having been a doctor for only twelve months, but the word *senior* had now been chucked into my job title. This was presumably to give patients a bit of confidence in the twenty-five-year-old about to take a scalpel to their abdomens. It was also the little morale boost I needed to stop myself jumping off the hospital roof when I first saw my new schedule. It would be pushing it to call it a promotion, though—it happens automatically after a year as a house officer.

I believe it's technically possible to fail the house-officer year and be required to repeat it, but I've never actually heard of that happening. By way of context, I count among my friends a house officer who slept with a patient in an on-call room and another who got distracted and prescribed penicillin instead of paracetamol to a patient with a penicillin allergy. They both sailed through it, so Christ knows what you have to do to actually fail.

Senior house officer is the point at which you decide what to specialize in. If you choose general practice, you remain in hospital for a couple of years, doing things like ER, internal medicine, and pediatrics, before moving to the community and being awarded your elbow patches and permanently raised eyebrow. If you choose hospital medicine, there are plenty of different roads you can stumble blindly down. If you fancy yourself as a surgeon, you can sign up to anything from colorectal surgery to cardiothoracic, neurosurgery to orthopedics. (Orthopedics is basically reserved for the med school's football team—it's barely more than sawing and nailing, and I suspect they don't "sign up" for it so much as dip their hands in ink and provide a palm print.) There are the various branches of general medicine if you don't like getting dirt under your nails—geriatrics,* cardiology, pulmonology, dermatology (which can be a revolting but relatively easy life;

---

* *Geriatrics* is now known as "care of the elderly." Presumably doctors want it to sound less clinical, less like a place where someone might actually expire and more like a luxury spa where you can get a mani-pedi while drinking something bright green from a smoothie-maker. Some hospitals have rebranded the specialty "care of the older patient" or "care of the older person"—I would suggest the more appropriate "care of the inevitable."

you can count the number of times you'd be woken up for a dermatological emergency on the fingers of one scaly, flaky hand), and so on. Plus there's a bunch of specialties that aren't quite medicine or surgery, like anesthesia, radiology, and obstetrics and gynecology.

I chose obs and gynae (as we call it; OB-GYN as you call it), or "brats and twats," as we charmingly referred to it at my medical school. I'd done my university thesis in the field, so I had a little bit of a head start as long as people only asked me questions about early neonatal outcome in the children of mothers with antiphospholipid syndrome, which somehow they never did. I liked that in obstetrics you ended up with twice the number of patients you started with, which is an unusually good batting average compared to other specialties. (I'm looking at you, geriatrics.) I also remembered being told by one of the registrars during my student placement that he'd chosen obs and gynae because it was easy. "Labor ward is literally four things: cesareans, forceps, vacuum extractions, and sewing up the mess you've made."*

I also liked the fact that it was a blend of medi-

---

* About a quarter of babies in the UK are delivered by cesarean section. Some are planned (elective) procedures for things like twins, breech babies, or previous cesareans. The rest are unplanned (emergency) cesareans for failure to progress in labor, fetal distress, and various other crises. If the baby gets stuck or distressed in the final furlong of a vaginal delivery, then you perform an "instrumental delivery" using either forceps—metal salad servers—or a suction cup attached to a vacuum cleaner. I wish I could say those descriptions were exaggerations.

cine and surgery; my house-officer jobs had proved I shouldn't really be majoring in either. It would give me a chance to work in infertility clinics and labor wards—what could be a better, more rewarding use of my training than delivering babies and helping couples who couldn't otherwise have them? Of course, the job would be difficult emotionally when things went wrong—not every stork has a happy landing—but unfortunately, the depth of the lows is the price you pay for the height of the highs.

There was also the fact that I'd ruled out every other specialty in quick succession: Too depressing. Too difficult. Too boring. Too revolting. Obs and gynae was the only one that excited me, a career I could genuinely look forward to.

In the event, it took me months to actually make up my mind, commit, and apply. I think the reason I hesitated was that I hadn't made any significant life decisions since I chose which medical school to go to as a teenager—and even that was mostly because I was impressed with the curly fries in the Student Union Hall. Age twenty-five was the first point I actually got to make an active decision in the Choose Your Own Adventure book of my life. I not only had to learn how to make a decision, but also ensure I made the right one.

You decide to pick up the forceps. Turn to page 41.

Monday, August 8, 2005

First week working on labor ward. Called in by the midwife because patient DH was feeling unwell shortly after delivering a healthy baby. Nobody likes a know-it-all, but it didn't take Poirot, Jessica Fletcher, and the entire occupancy of 221B Baker Street to work out the patient was probably "feeling unwell" because of the liters of blood cascading unnoticed out of her vagina. I pressed the emergency buzzer, hoped someone a bit more useful would appear, and unconvincingly assured the patient that everything was going to be fine while she continued to redecorate my legs with her blood volume.

The senior registrar ran in, performed a PV,* and removed a piece of placenta that was causing the issue.† Once it was coaxed out and the patient had a few units of blood replaced, she was absolutely fine.

I went to the changing rooms to get myself some fresh scrub pants. It's the third time in a week my boxers have been soaked in someone else's blood and I've had no option but to chuck them away and continue

---

* *PV* is a "per vagina" examination, and *PR* is a "per rectum" examination, so do always clarify when people tell you they work in PR.

† If there's anything left in the uterus after delivery—placenta, amniotic membranes, a Lego Darth Vader—the uterus can't contract back down properly, and this causes bleeding until the offending item is removed.

the shift commando. At fifteen pounds a pop for CKs, I think I'm running my job at a loss.

This time it had soaked through further than usual and I found myself washing blood off my cock. I'm not sure which is worse, the realization I could have caught HIV or the knowledge that none of my friends would ever believe *this* is how I got it.

Saturday, August 27, 2005

I'm accosted by a house officer to come and take a look at a postsurgical patient who hasn't passed urine in the last nine hours.* I tell the house officer that I haven't passed urine in the last *eleven* hours because of people like him wasting my time. His face crumples like a chips bag in a fat kid's fist and I instantly feel terrible for being mean to him—that was me a few months ago. I slink off to see the patient. The patient indeed has no urine output, but that's because the tubing from her catheter is trapped under the wheel of her bed and her bladder is the size of a Hoppity Hop ball. I stop feeling terrible.

---

* Doctors are obsessed with urine output, though not in the kind of way that would make you rethink going on a second date with them. It's how you tell if patients have low blood volume. This is particularly bad after surgery, as it could mean they're bleeding somewhere or that their kidneys are screwed, neither of which is great.

Monday, September 19, 2005

First vacuum-extraction delivery. I suddenly feel like an obstetrician—it's a pretty notional job title until you can, you know, actually extract a baby. My registrar, Lily, talks me through it gently, but I do it all myself and it feels fucking great.

"Congratulations, you did amazingly well there," says Lily.

"Thank you!" I reply, then realize she's actually talking to the mum.

Wednesday, September 21, 2005

Signing a stack of letters to GPs after gynae clinic when Ernie, one of the registrars—arrogant but funny with it—strides in to borrow an examination lamp. He peers over my shoulder. "You're going to get fired if you write that. Change it to *pus-like* or put a hyphen in there somewhere."

I look down at the offending phrase: *She has a pussy discharge.**

---

* At my next hospital, the gynecology ward was right next to the holding area they put patients in to await transport home, and the sign on the wall said

GYNAECOLOGY WARD

DISCHARGE LOUNGE

Wednesday, November 16, 2005

I glance at the notes before seeing an elderly gynae patient on ward rounds.

Good news: The physical therapists have finally been to see her.

Bad news: The entry reads, *Patient too drowsy to assess.*

I pop in. The patient is dead.

Tuesday, November 22, 2005

I've assisted registrars and consultants in fifteen cesareans now. On three or four occasions they've offered to let me operate while they teach me the steps, but every time, I've wimped out—I'm now the only SHO of the new cohort not to have lost my virginity, as Ernie is so keen on putting it.

Ernie doesn't give me any option today—he introduces me to the patient as the surgeon who's going to deliver her baby. And so I do. Cherry well and truly popped, and with a live audience. I cut through human skin for the first time, open up a uterus for the first time, and deliver a baby abdominally for the first time. I'd like to say it was an amazing experience, but I was concentrating far too hard on every step to actually take any of it in.

The cesarean takes a laborious fifty-five minutes[*] from start to end, and Ernie is remarkably patient with me. As I clean up the wound afterward, he points out that my incision was off by about ten degrees. He says to the patient, "You'll notice when you take the dressing off that we had to go in at a bit of an angle," which she somehow seems to accept without question—the miracle of motherhood sugaring that particular pill.

Ernie shows me how to write up the operation notes and debriefs me over coffee, stretching his virginity metaphor to within an inch of its life like he's some kind of sex pervert. Apparently, with practice, my technique will improve, it'll get less bloody and less nerve-racking, and eventually it'll all just start feeling like a boring routine. The anesthesiologist chimes in: "I wouldn't try and make your performance last any longer, though."

Sunday, December 25, 2005

Good news/bad news.

Good news: it's Christmas morning.[†]

---

[*] An uncomplicated cesarean should take only twenty to twenty-five minutes with the wind in the right direction.

[†] In the NHS, it's irrelevant that you worked the Christmas before, first because that was almost certainly in a different hospital and second because nobody gives the tiniest toss. There's a pecking order of those least likely to work at Christmas. First up is the doctor who organizes the schedule, followed by those with kids. Several rungs farther down this hierarchy comes me,

Bad news: I have to work on the labor ward.

Worse news: My phone goes off. It's my registrar. I didn't set my alarm and now they're wondering where the hell I am.

Even worse news: I'm asleep in my car. It takes me a while to establish where I am or why.

Good news: It seems I fell asleep after my shift last night and I'm already at work, in the hospital car park.

I leap out of the car, grab a quick shower, and then I'm good to go, a mere ten minutes late. I have eight missed calls from H and a text saying Merry Christmas, full stop, no kiss.

This year we're doing Christmas on my next day off, the sixth of January. "Just think how cheap the tinsel will be then!" was the only positive I could offer.

Wednesday, January 18, 2006

There are days when you get definitive confirmation of your place in the hospital hierarchy, and today's leveler was a cord prolapse.*

---

my childlessness burdening me with Christmas shifts practically every year. Despite having no great paternal yearnings (a feeling exacerbated by working on the labor ward), I seriously considered pretending to have children when I started a new job.

* *Cord prolapse* is when a loop or two of umbilical cord comes out through the vagina during labor, and unless this is right at the point of delivery, it means a very urgent cesarean. Fair enough that the cord got a little caught up in the moment and

I clamber onto the mattress behind the patient and assume the veterinary position, and the bed gets wheeled through to the OR. Another cesarean is just finishing up, so we wait in the anesthesia room for the time being. To keep the patient calm and make the situation seem less weird, we have a mundane chat about baby names, nappies, and maternity leave.

Her partner had nipped to the café downstairs for a few minutes just before things got this . . . intimate, so he missed all the drama. On his return, the midwife quickly brings him up to speed and gets him changed into scrubs so he can come to the OR for the cesarean. She leads him into the anesthesia room, where I'm kneeling, the vulva of the mother of his child halfway up my forearm. "Jesus Christ!" he says in a heavy Glasgow accent. The midwife remonstrates that she'd warned him I'd be holding the cord out of the way. "You did," he says, his eyes like dinner plates. "You didn't say he'd be wearing her like Kermit, though."

---

couldn't wait to make an appearance, like a firework exploding on the third of July, but if it gets cold, it goes into spasm, meaning there'll be no blood going to baby. It needs to be popped back into the vagina, and to keep pressure off the cord, the mother has to go up on all fours, resting on her knees and elbows, with the doctor standing behind until the moment she gets laid on her back for the cesarean. The doctor wears a very long glove that goes right up to the shoulder and is revoltingly called "the Gauntlet."

Tuesday, January 24, 2006

God has had the good sense to stay the hell away from my job, aside from a few *Holy fucks* and the odd *Jesus!* Today I meet with MM, a Jehovah's Witness, get her to sign a consent form for an open myomectomy.* It's a bloody type of operation, and we should have four units of crossmatched blood in the operating-theater fridge on standby.

The snag is, of course, that Jehovah's Witnesses refuse any blood transfusions because of their (fucking stupid) belief that blood contains the soul, and you shouldn't put someone else's soul into you. But it's a free country, so we respect everyone's (fucking stupid) values and wishes.

MM is bright, charming, and erudite, and we have a very interesting discussion. She agrees to have cell salvage† performed during the operation and I give her the specific consent form for refusing blood transfusion even if it's needed to save her life. It is a small possibil-

---

* A *myomectomy* is the removal of fibroids, benign swirls of growth in the muscle of the uterus that you take out using what is essentially a corkscrew.

† *Cell salvage* involves vacuuming up any blood that's lost during the operation, rather than swabbing it away, then running it through a machine that filters out any impurities (water used during the procedure, surgeon's sweat, bits of paint that have flaked off the ceiling). Should there be any need for a transfusion, the patient's own blood can be used—and some Witnesses believe this is in accordance with their teachings, as the blood stays within a closed circuit and isn't thought to have truly left the body. I know.

ity but a real one, even with cell salvage—numerous Jehovah's Witnesses have died because they declined blood products. She signs, though she admits part of the reason she's refusing is that her family would never speak to her again if she received blood. (Even more of an incentive to have a transfusion, if you ask me.)

Dr. Flitwick, my consultant, tells me that in his sepia-tinted, gung-ho version of "the good old days," they'd just ignore the form and plow ahead with a blood transfusion regardless, if needed; the patient would never find out, as she'd be under anesthesia. Happily, today's operation is gloriously uneventful and the cell-salvage machine stays in the corner of the room. I check on her back on the ward in the evening and on leafing through her notes, I see that her birthday is in two days and she'll most likely still be in hospital. I commiserate, despite the fact that I, too, will very likely be in a hospital for every single one of my birthdays until I'm too weak to blow out the candles, but she tells me that Jehovah's Witnesses don't celebrate birthdays or even receive presents. This is even more fucked up than the whole blood thing.

Thursday, January 26, 2006

Moral maze. On ward rounds, Ernie is talking to a very well-spoken woman in her thirties, basically a younger, posher version of the Queen. She's ready to go home after an emergency admission a few days ago with ovarian torsion.* He books her for follow-up in the clinic in six weeks and tells her not to drive for three weeks. "Oh, for heaven's sake!" she says to Ernie. "The bloody thing's in the car park here. Why don't *you* just drive it until I see you in clinic?" Ernie is about to say no, that's insane, until she complicates matters by pulling a set of Bentley keys from her handbag. Anyway, Ernie currently drives a Bentley Continental GT.

Friday, January 27, 2006

I've been visiting Baby L on SCBU† for three months now—it's become part of my routine before I head home, and it's nice to see a familiar face, even if it's through the glass of an incubator wall.‡ His mum

---

* *Ovarian torsion* is where the ovary twists round on itself and cuts off its blood supply; if not operated on very quickly, it goes black and dies. And if not operated on at all, the entire patient becomes septic, then goes black and dies.

† *SCBU* (pronounced "Scaboo") is the Special Care Baby Unit; *NICU* is the Neonatal Intensive Care Unit; *PICU* is the Pediatric Intensive Care Unit; and *PIKACHU* is a type of Pokémon.

‡ Something very unsatisfying about house-officer jobs was the way you never found out the end of the story; every patient's box set was missing the final DVD. A patient would come in with pneumonia, you'd get him well enough to go home, and then he was gone—he could live another fifteen years, die on the bus home, or anything in between, and you'd almost certainly never know. Extreme nosiness aside, I always felt like it might have been useful to find out if our management plans were any use. I liked that obstetrics played out much quicker; you got to watch right through to the credits, and by reflecting

was admitted on my second Saturday on the job, twenty-six weeks into her first pregnancy, with a blistering headache that, it quickly transpired, was severe early-onset preeclampsia.* She was stabilized and we delivered Baby L on the Sunday; I assisted the consultant in the C-section. Mum ended up spending a few days in intensive care—so we definitely couldn't have waited any longer before delivering—and baby came out a tiny scrap of a thing, weighing in at just over a jar of jam.

Neonatologists make obstetricians look like orthopedic surgeons; they're so academic, so meticulous, defying God and nature to make these babies pull through. As recently as 1970, this baby would have

---

back on your decisions in the context of these outcomes, you could learn and improve as a doctor. And so, if a baby went to SCBU, I made a point of popping by to see how it was doing.

* *Preeclampsia* is a disorder of pregnancy that can affect most organs of the mum's body, causing liver and kidney damage, swelling of the brain, fluid in the lungs, and platelet problems, as well as problems with the baby's growth and well-being. It ultimately progresses to eclampsia—life-threatening seizures. Most cases of preeclampsia are mild, but every pregnant patient has her blood pressure and urine protein measured at each visit in order to pick up the condition at an early stage. The only cure for preeclampsia is delivering the placenta (and necessarily the baby first). The vast majority of preeclamptic patients end up just being monitored throughout pregnancy, taking some tablets to reduce their blood pressure or having labor induced a week or two early. Some patients, however, develop the condition severely and much earlier in pregnancy, leading to the painful decision to deliver the baby prematurely to prevent terrible consequences for both mother and child.

had chances of survival under 10 percent, but today the odds are over 90 percent. After twelve weeks of neonatology magic, he's gone from a transparent-skinned shrew attached to a dozen tubes and wires to a proper screaming, vomiting, sleeping little baby, and he's getting discharged home this afternoon.

I should be delighted he's going home—and I am, of course, that's our entire raison d'être—but I'm going to miss seeing my little pal every couple of days.

I buy the mum the least ghastly card they have in the hospital shop, say how pleased I am their story had a happy ending and ask her to maybe text me a picture of him every so often, then leave the card with the pediatric nurses to pass on. Yes, it's probably against GMC regulations and hospital protocol and violates all sorts of small print, guidelines, and best practices, but I'm prepared to go down for this one.*

Thursday, February 2, 2006

Signing letters to GPs in the gynae office.

Dear Doctor,

I saw XA in clinic with her husband, Sam, Esther Sugar, and their two children . . .

---

* And she did text me.

A moment while I try to remember the appointment. Who of these three were the children's parents? I feel I should know who Esther is—why the full name? Is she famous? A reality-TV star, maybe? As it turns out, Esther wasn't there at all.

Two months ago, the trust laid off almost all the hospital secretaries and replaced them with a new computer system. The first key difference is that, rather than giving your Dictaphone tapes to the secretaries, you now dictate straight onto your clinic computer, which chooses to either upload your audio and send it abroad to the secretarial equivalent of a sweatshop or instantly delete it without a trace. The second key difference is that the quality of the transcription would suggest the back end of the system involves two tin cans, a length of string, and a lemur who's been trained to type. We're not to worry about that, though; the main thing is all the money the trust is saving by sacking so many long-serving, hardworking members of staff who adored the hospital. The one advantage of this system is that you can listen back to your original audio when reviewing documents. I press Play.

Dear Doctor,

I saw XA in clinic with her husband, Sam (S for sugar), and their two children.

I'm confident this takes me to the top of the leaderboard in departmental-dictation fuckups, unseating

The patient has known analogies (no known allergies).

Wednesday, March 22, 2006

Three a.m. attendance at labor-ward triage. Patient RO is twenty-five years old and thirty weeks into her first pregnancy. She complains of a large number of painless spots on her tongue. Diagnosis: taste buds.

Monday, April 3, 2006

It's two a.m. and there's not much doing on labor ward so I slope off to the on-call room to catch up on some personal admin (Adamin?) and stare at Facebook for a bit. I comment on how cute a friend's latest ugly baby looks, which I can do very convincingly, as I spend a large proportion of my working day doing the same thing to total strangers. For me, the true miracle of childbirth is that smart, rational people with jobs and the ability to vote look at these half-melted fleshy blobs, their heads misshapen from being squeezed through a pelvis, covered in five types of horrendous gunk, looking like they've spent a good two hours rolling around on top of a deep-pan pizza, and honestly believe they look beautiful. It's Darwinism in action, an irrational love for your progeny. The same hardwired desire to keep the species going that sees a woman come back to the labor ward for round two eighteen months after the irreparable destruction of her perineum.

The other miracle of childbirth is that I can put metal forceps on a baby's head and lean backward—applying fifty pounds of traction force on it, generally getting a sweat on—and the baby comes out absolutely fine rather than, as you might expect, decapitated. Once the baby's born, every new mother obsesses over keeping the head straight with a cradled hand. If photographs could talk, *Careful of his neck!* is the shriek you'd hear over any picture of a childless relative posing with a newborn. But I'm pretty sure you could carry it by its head and it'd be totally okay.*

I'm just going through exes' profiles to check if they're overweight and colossally miserable without me when I see a post pop up from Simon, a school friend's younger brother. He's twenty-two, and even though I've spoken to him only twice, a decade ago, this is Facebook, where everyone's your friend. It's simple and devastatingly effective. Four words: *Goodbye, everyone. I'm done.*

I realize I'm probably the only person to be reading this at two thirty a.m. on a Monday, so I send him a private message to ask if he's okay. I say I'm awake, remind him I'm a doctor, and give him my mobile number. I'm scrolling through my phone to see if I have his brother's number when Simon rings. He's an

---

* This is not medical advice.

absolute mess; drunk, crying. He's just split up with his girlfriend.

I'm actually no better trained to counsel him than I am to talk him through replacing a gearbox or laying a parquet floor, but he assumes I am, and that's good enough for both of us. Two (miraculously bleep-free) hours later and we've had a good chat. He's going to get a cab to his mum's, then make an emergency appointment with his GP in the morning. I feel the same weird endorphin rush I get after dealing with any medical emergency—exhaustion plus exhilaration and the vague feeling of having done a "good thing" (like how you'd feel after a 10k charity run). It's likely I've made a bigger difference to Simon than to any of my patients tonight.

I answer a bleep and head to the labor ward to see a woman at thirty weeks who's decided she needs her eczema evaluated at five a.m. "I thought it would be quieter now than in the morning," she says.

Monday, April 10, 2006

Referral from an SHO in the ER—a patient has some kind of warty vulval growth. I ask him if he can describe it a bit more. "Like cauliflower florets, mate. Actually, what with the discharge, it's more like broccoli."

H did not enjoy this story over dinner.

Friday, April 21, 2006

Ron is having a minor knee op next week and wants me to reassure him that he's not going to die during the anesthesia, reassurance that I'm underqualified yet perfectly happy to give him.

He also asks if sometimes the anesthesia doesn't work, so I tell him a story from earlier this year:

"So, there are two main drugs that anesthesiologists give. First, a paralytic, so that the surgeon can have a proper fiddle-around. With the body completely paralyzed, you can't breathe unassisted, which is why you get hooked up to a ventilator during the procedure. The second drug's a cloudy fluid called propofol that makes you unconscious, so you're asleep throughout the procedure.

"Now imagine that your anesthesiologist accidentally grabs the wrong cloudy fluid off his trolley and injects you with an antibiotic instead of propofol. You're lying on an operating table, totally paralyzed, but without the propofol you're entirely awake, able to hear everything that's being said, able to feel the surgeon cleaning you up with antiseptic, and you have no way of alerting anyone that something's gone horribly wrong. You silently scream as his scalpel cuts through your skin—a worse, more searing pain than you've ever experienced in your life . . . "Ron's expression looks like it's been drawn on by Edvard Munch. "But I'm sure you'll be just fine!"

Tuesday, June 6, 2006

Called to see a patient in the ER. She had a medical termination of pregnancy a couple of days ago and is in absolute agony. I don't quite know what the matter is, but something is definitely up—I admit her to the ward for pain relief and senior review. Ernie examines her.

"She's having cramping pains. Scan before her MTOP showed an intrauterine pregnancy. Normal. Send her home."

I try to justify my admission—surely this is way too much pain? She's on morphine!

"Only because you prescribed her morphine."

No one is in pain like this with an MTOP, though, I say.

"How do *you* know her pain threshold?" comes the no-nonsense reply. "Maybe she's like this when she stubs her toe as well."

I venture that something weird is going on here, and he dismisses me.

"If you hear hooves clip-clopping outside your bedroom window, it *could* be a zebra. But when you take a look, it will almost always turn out to be a horse." He tells me I can prescribe her some antibiotics just in case there's an infection brewing, but she still needs to go home.

The bleep from the ward saying that the patient had deteriorated would ideally have come at that exact moment. Instead, it came a few hours later, but the result was the same: assisting Ernie in the operating theater to remove an ectopic pregnancy* and a metric fuckton of blood from her pelvis. The scan she'd had before her termination was dangerously wrong.

The patient is now fine and back on the ward. Ernie hasn't apologized to me, as that would require him to change his entire personality. I'm currently on Amazon, ordering him a key ring in the shape of a zebra.

Monday, June 12, 2006

Counseling a patient that weight loss would help control her PCOS,† I refer her to the dietician and ask her about exercise. Just because something is obvious to me does not mean it's obvious to the patient—it feels

---

* An *ectopic pregnancy* is when an embryo attaches in the wrong place, most frequently in a fallopian tube. Left untreated, it will eventually rupture, and this is the most common cause of death in women in the first three months of pregnancy. Every woman with pain and a positive pregnancy test is considered to have an ectopic until proven otherwise by a scan. In this case, the scanner had mistakenly interpreted an ectopic pregnancy as an intrauterine one.

† *Polycystic ovarian syndrome (PCOS)* is the most common endocrine condition in women, affecting between one in five and one in twenty females, depending on how the disorder is defined, which will have changed another three or four times between me writing this and you reading it. PCOS can cause problems with fertility, increased body hair, and menstrual disturbances.

like knocking on the door of a blazing building to tell the owner his house is on fire, but occasionally it does make a difference. Steeling myself for the predictable answer about a lack of time, I offer: "It might help you to join a gym?"

"I'm a member of one already" comes the reply. "But I haven't been in about three thousand pounds."

Monday, June 19, 2006

Called to urgently assess a patient on the prenatal-care ward. Patient ES is having her labor induced for post-maturity.[*] The concerned midwife leads me to a toilet on the ward; the patient has just opened her bowels, and the pan looks like the Body Shop has released a horrific new red-and-brown bath bomb. It doesn't au-gur well for either the cleaners' tea break or the patient herself.

I examine her to make sure the bleeding isn't vagi-nal, which it isn't, and am pleased to see the baby looks fine on the CTG.[†] The rectal examination was totally

---

[*] Much like your drunk mate insisting you go on to one more club even though she's already got vomit in her hair, pregnan-cies sometimes keep going longer than is wise. After forty-two weeks, the placenta can start to give up the ghost, so we induce labor before mums get to that point, the first step being a tablet or gel such as Prostin inserted vaginally.

[†] The *cardiotocograph*, known as the CTG or "trace," is a moni-tor strapped to the mum during labor that measures and con-tinuously records contractions and the baby's heart rate. The

normal, the patient says she's never had anything like this before and has no other symptoms. I send off blood, crossmatch her, put up some fluids, and refer her urgently to gastro. I also google whether Prostin can cause massive gastrointestinal bleeding. There's no history of it happening before, so this would be the first case—I idly wonder whether they'll name the syndrome after me. I was rather hoping Kay syndrome might be a more glamorous discovery than someone shitting herself inside out during induction of labor, but perhaps it's a price worth paying for immortalization in the textbooks.

The gastro consultant appears before I've finished writing up my notes, and after a quick chat and another lubricated finger, she's wheeled off for a colonoscopy. Happily, all looks normal and there's no evidence of recent bleeding. A bit of further questioning, and the consultant comes up with the diagnosis; he bleeps to let me know.

The nightmare in the toilet bowl I'd witnessed was in fact the rather damning evidence of the two large jars of pickled beetroot that ES had inexplicably taken it upon herself to eat the night before. Next time I want to refer him someone's bowel movement, the consultant "respectfully" asks that I taste it first.

---

readout is generally described as either a "reassuring trace" or a "non-reassuring trace."

Tuesday, June 20, 2006

Our computer system has been upgraded and, as happens eleven times out of ten when the hospital tries to make life easier, they've made everything much more complicated. It certainly looks much whizzier (and less like an MS-DOS program from school), but they've not actually fixed any of the massive clunking problems with the software; they've just slapped an interface on top of it. It's the equivalent of treating skin cancer by putting makeup over the lesion. Actually, it's worse than that. This glossy interface uses so much of the exhausted system's resources that it's now slowed to a nearly unusable crawl. It's like treating skin cancer with some makeup that the patient has an extreme allergic reaction to.

The blood tests now all live in a drop-down menu, and ordering one involves scrolling down an alphabetical list of every test any doctor has ever ordered in the history of humanity. To get down to *vitamin B*$_{12}$ takes three minutes and seventeen seconds. And if you press the letter *V* rather than wading down there manually, the system crashes so badly you have to unplug the computer and all but use a soldering iron to get it working again. Ninety-nine percent of the time we order the same dozen tests, and yet, rather than being prioritized at the top of the list (even the Southwest Airlines website knows to put the UK and US above Albania and Azerbaijan), they're scattered throughout a billion tests I've never heard of or requested. Who knew there were three different lab tests for serum selenium? As a result, there's a very narrow window of anemic patients I will now order vitamin B_{12} levels for. If you're only mildly anemic I'm not wasting the day with my finger pressing on the down arrow for three minutes. And if you're severely anemic, I won't order it because you'll probably be dead by the time I've done so.

Friday, July 21, 2006

Bleeped to the gynae ward at five a.m. to write a discharge summary for a patient due to go home in the morning. It should have been done yesterday by her own SHO and there's no reason for me to be doing it, but if I don't do it now it will delay the patient's discharge. I sit down and get on with it—it's fairly mindless work so it gives me a bit of time to plot some appropriate revenge act on the SHO in question. On my way out, I notice the light is on in patient CR's side room, so I pop my head in to check if everything's okay.

I admitted her from the ER last week with tense ascites* and the suspicion of an ovarian mass. I've been on nights since and not kept up with what's happened. She tells me. "Suspicion of an ovarian mass" has be-

---

* *Ascites* is fluid in the abdomen and almost always very bad news.

come a diagnosis of ovarian cancer has become confirmation of widespread metastases has become talk of a few months left. When I saw her in the ER, despite my obvious suspicions, I didn't say the word *cancer*—I was taught that if you say that word even in passing, that's all a patient remembers. Doesn't matter what else you do; utter the C-word just once and you've basically walked into the cubicle and said nothing but "Cancer cancer cancer cancer cancer" for half an hour. And not that you'd ever want *any* patient to have cancer, of course, but I really, *really* didn't want her to. She was friendly, funny, chatty—despite the liters of fluid in her abdomen splinting her breathing—we were like two long-lost pals finding themselves next to each other at a bus stop and catching up on all our years apart. Her son has a place at med school; her daughter is at the same school my sister went to; she recognized my socks were Duchamp. I stuck in a Bonanno catheter to take off the fluid and admitted her to the ward for the day team to investigate.

And now she's telling me what they found. She bursts into tears, and out come all the *will nevers*, the crushing realization that *forever* is just a word on the front of Valentine's cards. Her son will graduate from medical school—she won't be there. Her daughter will get married—she won't be able to help with the table plan or throw confetti. She'll never meet her grandchildren. Her husband will never get over it. "He doesn't even know how to work the thermostat!" She laughs, so I laugh. I really don't know what to say. I want to lie and tell her everything's going to be fine, but we both know that it won't. I hug her. I've never hugged a patient before—in fact, I think I've hugged a grand total of five people, and one of my parents isn't even on that list—but I don't know what else to do.

We talk about boring, practical things, rational concerns, irrational concerns, and I can see from her eyes it's helping her. It suddenly strikes me that I'm almost certainly the first person she's opened up to about all this, the only one she's been totally honest with. It's a strange privilege, an honor I didn't ask for.

The other thing I realize is that none of her many, many concerns are about herself; it's all about the kids, her husband, her sister, her friends. Maybe that's the definition of a good person.

We had a patient in obstetrics a couple of months ago who was diagnosed with metastatic breast cancer during pregnancy and was advised to deliver at thirty-two weeks so she could start treatment but waited until thirty-seven weeks to give her baby the absolute best possible chance. She died after a fortnight spent with her baby—who knows whether starting treatment a month sooner would have made any difference. Probably not.

And now I'm sitting with a woman who's asking me if she should have her ashes scattered on the Scilly Isles. It's her favorite spot, but she doesn't want it to be a sad place for her family once she's gone. The undiluted selflessness of someone fully aware of what her absence will do to those she leaves behind. My bleeper goes off—it's the morning SHO asking for handover. I've spent two hours in this room, the longest I've ever spent with a patient who wasn't under anesthesia. On the way home I phone my mum to tell her I love her.

3

Senior House Officer—Post Two

Sometime during my early years as an SHO, I remember watching a documentary about Shaolin kung fu masters. They train for a decade or more in a remote temple, waking up at five a.m. and only stopping at midnight, submitting themselves to a life of celibacy, devoid of material possessions. I couldn't help but feel it didn't sound that bad—at least they didn't have to uproot their lives every year and go to a completely different temple.

NHS deaneries, who are responsible for postgraduate medical training, move doctors to different hospitals every six or twelve months to ensure they learn from a broad range of consultants, which I guess makes sense. Unfortunately, each deanery covers a fairly large geographical area, and you get randomly allocated to units throughout that region. For example, one such deanery is called Scotland. You know

Scotland, that—what would you call it . . . oh, yes—entire *country* measuring over thirty thousand square miles. If you're deciding where to buy your first house, it's rather difficult to choose a location that's handy for all of Scotland. Even if you were insane enough to put yourself through a property transaction once or twice a year, it would be fairly tricky, as the deaneries limit relocation costs to a princely zero pounds.

So while all my friends in sensible careers were getting mortgages and puppies, H and I were taking on yearlong rental contracts and living somewhere mutually inconvenient roughly halfway between our two workplaces. It was yet another item on the list of ways my job was inflicting collateral damage on H—medical widow, post-shift counselor, and now nomad.

I remember once phoning round all the various utility companies about our change of address (I think as penance because I couldn't take the day off work to help with the move) and the home-insurance people asked a standard question about the number of nights the property is left empty. I realized that if I lived alone, the policy would be invalid, as it would technically be considered an "unoccupied property."

Despite the hours, I'd really enjoyed my first year in obs and gynae—I'd made the right choice. I'd gone from a tottering Bambi, terrified every time the bleeper went off, to, if not a graceful roebuck, then at least someone who could do a decent impression of one. I now had a bit of self-belief that I could deal with the emergency behind each delivery-room door, mostly thanks to working in a hospital with seniors who were invested in my development as a doctor.

When the deanery rolled the dice for the second time, however, I found myself in a much more old-fashioned hospital. If you describe a grandparent as being *old-fashioned*, it's a euphemism for "casually racist." In a hospital setting, it means "unsupportive." You're on your own.

I'd gone from a nursery slope straight to a Schumacher-splattering black run where the senior doctors took the now largely extinct approach of "see one, do one, teach one": You've watched someone remove a fallopian tube or scan an ovary, so that's you, fully trained up. You'd be forgiven for thinking this was a horrible nightmare. As it turned out, at this hospital, it was often the best-case scenario, "see one" frequently getting skipped over, like foreplay in a nightclub-restroom tryst.

Nowadays, YouTube instructional videos can show you anything from how to repair an ingrown toenail to how to separate conjoined twins.* Back in 2006, you had to follow a list of printed instructions in a textbook. To add to the fun, you'd have to memorize these generally quite complicated steps (think assembling a car rather than an Ikea dresser) before you saw the patient. How much confidence would you have in someone staring at your genitals with a scalpel in one hand and a manual in the other? I rapidly learned to

---

* Please don't attempt either.

maintain an air of absolute confidence no matter how frantically my legs were paddling under the water. In summary, never play poker with me. Although do bear me in mind if you're struggling with your some-assembly-required furniture.

Because I spent the vast proportion of my waking hours at work and because the deep end was so very deep, I learned a lot during my second SHO post and did so very quickly. The old-fashioned method might not be any fun, but it definitely works. Those Shaolin bastards were basically at holiday camp.

Wednesday, August 2, 2006

It's Black Wednesday[*] and I have started at St. Agatha's. It is an established fact that hospital death rates go up on Black Wednesday. Knowing this really takes the pressure off, so I'm not trying very hard.

Thursday, August 10, 2006

Seeing a mother in clinic six weeks after a traumatic delivery. All is now well, but something is clearly trou-

---

[*] All junior doctors change hospitals on exactly the same day every six or twelve months, a day known as Black Wednesday. You might think it would be a terrible idea to exchange all your Scrabble tiles in one go and expect the hospital to run exactly as it did the day before, and you'd be quite right.

bling her. I ask her what's up and she breaks down in tears—she thinks the baby has a brain tumor and asks me to have a look. It's very much not my department[*] but one look at the mother's collapsed face tells me that now perhaps wouldn't be the best time to play the unhelpful station assistant at a ticket window and advise she should see her GP. I examine the child and hope that whatever she's concerned about is within the limited parameters of my pediatric knowledge.

She shows me a hard swelling on the back of baby's head. My ship has somehow come in and I can confidently announce that this is baby's occipital protuberance, which is a completely normal part of the skull. Look, there it is on your other kid's head! There it is on your head!

"Oh my God," she cries, the tears still streaking her face, eyes darting from her baby to her three-year-old and back again, like she's watching the Wimbledon final. "It's hereditary."

---

[*] Parents seem to think obstetricians are wise owls with expert knowledge of infants, but this couldn't be farther from the truth. We know the square root of fuck all about them save for a few half-remembered semi-facts from medical school. Once babies are no longer umbilically attached to their mothers, we hand them over and don't deal with them again until they're old enough to procreate.

Monday, August 14, 2006

My schedule involves scanning in the early pregnancy unit once a fortnight. Today, having never so much as *seen* a scan like this performed before, I had to single-shaking-handedly run a clinic of twenty patients, peering at four-millimeter lumps of cells using a trans-vaginal probe.[*]

I asked (begged) a registrar to give me a quick demo, and he had time to see one patient with me before he dashed off to the OR. My SHO colleague on the afternoon shift had never done it before either, so I passed on my new skill by scanning her first patient for her. See one, do twenty, teach one.

Wednesday, August 16, 2006

Just out of a delivery, my slickest vacuum extraction yet. The midwife told me afterward she assumed I was a registrar (although she *is* known as Dangerous Dawn, so I'm not going to put vast quantities of stock in that).

A phone call from Mum to say my sister Sophie's got into med school. I send Soph a text with huge con-

---

[*] This sounds like a high-speed train service in the Caucasus but is considerably less sophisticated. You look inside the uterus with an ultrasound stick to decide if a pregnancy is viable, miscarrying, or ectopic. Misdiagnosis can see you the wrong side of a negligence/manslaughter charge.

gratulations, then a picture of me thumbs-upping in scrubs (cropped above the spatter-zone) and You in six years' time!

Had the call come at the end of the shift, my text would have read, Run like the fucking wind.

Monday, August 21, 2006

I've been carrying a package-delivery company's *Sorry you were out* notice around with me for over a fortnight. I keep taking it out and looking at it meaningfully like it's a photograph of my firstborn or some long-dead childhood sweetheart, pathetically rereading the facility's hours on the off chance that they will magically alter before my eyes. They do not.

I wouldn't have time to get there and back on my lunch hour, even if I had a lunch hour, which of course I don't, but I've been holding on to a glimmer of hope that I might knock off work early one day—if the hospital burned down, say, or nuclear war was declared. Today I start a week of nights, so I nip off to collect the parcel. Unfortunately, it turns out they hold on to items for only eighteen days, every one of which I've been at work, so it's been returned to sender.

Long story short, H won't be getting a birthday present tomorrow.

Thursday, September 14, 2006

Patient CW on the prenatal-care ward needs some imaging done of her lungs, so I book her for an MRI and go through the checklist.* She is in fact ineligible for an MRI, having had a small but powerful magnet implanted in the pulp of her right index finger a few years ago.

Apparently there had been a limited trend for this, performed by tattoo artists and intended to give the recipients an "extra sense"—an otherworldly awareness of metal objects around them, like a kind of vibrating aura (her words) or a slightly low-rent X-Man (my words).

Her sales pitch needs work, to be honest. It turned out not to be the mystical, ethereal experience she had been looking for but a regal pain in the arse—she tells me it's become infected a number of times, and going

---

* Ordinarily you'd do a CT scan, but we try to avoid those in pregnancy as they involve a large quantity of X-ray exposure, and anyone who's stayed up for the late-night horror movie can tell you that radiation plus baby is not a good idea. I've had the mechanism of MRIs explained to me any number of times and I'm still none the wiser, but no X-rays are involved; images are obtained using a combination of protons, magic, and an enormous fucking magnet. And I mean enormous, the size and weight of a one-bedroom flat. The MRI checklist asks if the patient's got a metal heart valve (it would tear out of her now-dead chest at eighty miles an hour and splat onto the machine) or worked in a metal factory (tiny bits of metal would have found their way into her eyes, making both eyeballs explode when she opened the door to the MRI suite).

through airport security is now a living hell. I briefly toy with asking her to brush past my colleague Cormac to either confirm or refute the rumor that he has a Prince Albert,* but she says the implant has recently become either dislodged or demagnetized and now she barely feels a thing except for a lump in her finger. She wants to have the magnet removed, in fact, but the scar tissue that will have formed around it makes it a slightly involved operation and one not covered on the NHS. I book her for a CT scan—she can wear a lead apron and there'll be very little radiation exposure for the baby. Although if I'd gone ahead and booked her for an MRI, I'd have saved her the cost of that private operation.

Sunday, September 17, 2006

Either the printer has gone insane or one of the receptionists has—huge quantities of paper have engulfed the nursing station. Everyone in sight has collected around the machine to try and fix it, all doing exactly the same thing—jabbing random buttons to absolutely zero effect.

Pages are cascading out of the printer and onto the

---

* The already-close-to-zero appeal of a genital piercing instantly evaporated for me when, as a house officer, I saw a patient present with an injury caused by a ring getting ripped out during sex. This happens frequently enough that urologists have a term for it: *Prince Albert's revenge.*

labor-ward floor. I pick one up—they're patient iden-
tification stickers for a neonate, to go on notes, wrist-
bands, et cetera. For the rest of the day, we all check
our shoes and backs in paranoia, just in case a stray
one has become attached—this is one label nobody
wants to be walking around with, since a slightly unfortunate surname means that every sticker says BABY
RAPER.

Wednesday, September 27, 2006

I'm off sick for the first time since graduating. Work
wasn't exactly sympathetic.

"Oh, for fuck's sake," spat my registrar when I
rang in. "Can't you just come in for the morning?"
I explained I had quite bad food poisoning and was
in some kind of gastrointestinal meltdown. "Fine,"
he said with the kind of weary, simmering passive-
aggression I normally get only at home. "But phone
around and find someone who's on leave to cover you."

I'm pretty sure this isn't the protocol at Google or
General Motors or even at grocery stores. Is there a
single other workplace where you'd conceivably be
asked to arrange your own sickness cover? The North
Korean army, maybe? I wonder what level of illness
would stop it from being my responsibility. Broken
pelvis? Lymphoma? Or just when I was intubated in
the ICU and denied the power of speech?

Luckily, I could manage to force out a few words

between bouts of vomiting (if not between bouts of diarrhea), so I was able to organize a stand-in. I didn't explain what I was doing during the call—it probably sounded like I'd gone paintballing. And I now owe her a shift in return, so it's not even sick *leave*.

I'd always suspected if I ended up calling in sick it would be work that caused it. My money would have been on some form of emotional collapse, maybe renal failure from dehydration, getting beaten up by an angry relative, or smashing my car into a tree after a sleep-deprived night shift. As it happens, it was an altogether stealthier assassin—a portion of noxious homemade moussaka from a laboring patient's mother. I can be fairly sure that was the culprit; it was the only thing I'd managed to eat all day. There should be a saying about Greeks bearing gifts, I thought, shitting through the eye of a hypodermic needle, the taste of bile and faint tinge of aubergine in my throat.

Saturday, September 30, 2006

Evaluating a woman in triage, who just arrived huffing and puffing away in labor. I ask how frequently the contractions are coming and the husband tells me they're three to four times every ten minutes, lasting up to a minute each. I explain I'll need to do an internal examination to assess how far dilated* she is.

The husband tells me he checked before they left home and she was at six centimeters. Most dads-to-be don't peek under the hood so I ask him if he's a physician. No, he tells me, he's a plasterer, but "I know what a centimeter is, mate." I examine the patient and agree with his findings, which makes him more competent than most of my colleagues.

Saturday, October 7, 2006

I've now spent six months being Simon's on-call mental-health help line since that first Facebook post—any time he's having worrying thoughts, I've told him he can ring me, and he does. I've also told him repeatedly to engage more formally with mental-health services, but he's not so keen on listening to that bit. Aside from the fact it's a bit overwhelming to now have a second bleep threatening to go off with

---

* The contractions of the womb make its neck, or cervix, go from closed before labor starts to full (ten centimeters) dilation at the end of labor, at which point baby can make its grand entrance. The first few centimeters of dilation can take an extremely long time, so women aren't generally admitted to the labor ward until they're at least three centimeters dilated—like a strange nightclub you can't get into until you've had two gloved fingers in your vagina. Actually, there's probably one of those in Soho already.

bad news any minute, I suspect he can get better help from someone who didn't have to panic-google *What to say to someone who's suicidal*. But it seems I'm better than nothing—at the very least, he's still alive.

The most stressful part is discovering I've missed a call from him—if I call back too late and he's done himself in, does that make it my fault, like I'm the one who kicked away the chair? I suppose it doesn't, but that's how you feel as a doctor and probably why I'm in this situation to begin with. If you're the first to notice someone else's patient is breathing strangely or has abnormal blood tests, it's your responsibility to deal with it, or at least ensure someone else does. I'm pretty sure heating engineers don't feel the same way about every kaput boiler they encounter. The difference is obviously the whole life-and-death thing, which is what separates this job from all others and makes it so unfathomable to people on the outside.

I call Simon back after a cesarean this evening. I've got my counseling sessions down to about twenty minutes—it's just a case of listening, being sympathetic, and reassuring him the feelings will pass. He must realize we have the same chat every time, but it clearly doesn't matter—he just wants to know there's someone out there who cares. And actually, that's a very large part of what being a doctor is.

Monday, October 9, 2006

Today crossed the line from everyday patient idiocy to me checking the room for *Punk'd*'s hidden cameras. After a lengthy discussion with a patient's husband about how absolutely no condoms fit him, I establish he's pulling them right down over his balls.

Tuesday, October 10, 2006

I missed what the argument was about, but a woman storms out of gynae outpatient clinic screaming at the nurse, "I pay your salary! I pay your salary!" The nurse yells back, "Can I have a raise, then?"

Monday, October 23, 2006

Asked to come to the ER to assess a gentleman in his seventies. I check to see if the ER doctor realizes he's bleeped gynecology; evaluating a man would be rather pushing my remit. It's complicated, apparently; he'll explain when I get down there.

I meet patient NS, a Sikh gentleman who speaks no English at all. He is on holiday, visiting family, and has been unhelpfully accompanied to the hospital by a relative who also speaks no English. His history is therefore taken with the assistance of a telephone-interpreter service—in this instance, a Punjabi translator is on the line and the phone is passed back and forth. This particular interpreter may have rather fudged his CV—he seems to be able to speak only slightly more Punjabi than someone who can't speak any Punjabi whatsoever.

The stoic ER staff have been making glacial progress using the interpreter, and they relay what they've established: the patient is bleeding from "down below," has been doing so for the past week, and—crucially to my attendance—is a hermaphrodite.* I tell the ER doctor that I sincerely doubt this elderly bearded man is part of the intersex community and ask to speak to the interpreter.

"Can you ask if the patient has a womb?" The phone gets passed back, and the patient starts to repeat a word to us very loudly and angrily in Punjabi. The patient furiously unbuttons his shirt to reveal a Port-a-Cath†—our eureka moment. In unison we all say, "Hemophiliac!" and I leave them to deal with his rectal bleed.

---

* *Hermaphroditism* is a very rare intersex disorder in which an individual possesses both testicular and ovarian tissue. It's named after the Greek legend of Hermaphroditus, who was said to be both male and female. He/she was the son/daughter of Hermes and Aphrodite, who it must be said had a pretty lazy system for naming their children.

† A *Port-a-Cath* is a device that sits under the skin to allow easy injection of drugs and taking of blood for people who need it done frequently.

Tuesday, October 31, 2006

Moral maze. In the labor-ward dressing rooms after a long shift. I'm leaving at ten p.m. rather than eight p.m., thanks to a major obstetric hemorrhage that ended up back in the operating theater. I'm meant to be going to a Halloween party, but now I don't have time to go home and pick up my costume. However, I am currently dressed in scrubs and spattered head to toe in blood. Would it be *so* wrong?

Saturday, November 4, 2006

Get bleeped to see a postpartum patient at 1:00 a.m. The OR staff relay to the bleeping midwife that I'm in the middle of a cesarean. I get bleeped again at 1:15 a.m. (still doing the section) and 1:30 a.m. (writing up my operation notes). Eventually, I head off to assess the patient. The big emergency? She's going home in the morning and wants to have her passport application countersigned by a doctor while she's still in here.

Wednesday, November 15, 2006

I have signed up for the MRCOG* part one exam. A textbook advises me to try a past exam before I start

---

* Member of the Royal College of Obstetricians and

studying—"You might be pleasantly surprised how much you already know!" I attempt one.

March 1997, Paper 1, Question 1
True or false? Chromaffin cells:

A. Are innervated by preganglionic sympathetic nerve fibers
B. Are present in the adrenal cortex
C. Are derived from neuro-ectoderm
D. Can decarboxylate amino acids
E. Are present in celiac ganglia

Aside from the fact that I know what less than half of these words mean (and most of the ones I do know are prepositions), I can't help wondering how it's relevant to my baby-delivering abilities. But if it's what my insane demonic overlords want me to know, who am I to argue?

Another textbook cheerily informs me that it's quite possible to prepare for MRCOG part one in just six months "with an hour or two's study every evening." It's one of those phrases that is intended to be reassuring but has the opposite effect, like "It's only a small tumor" or "Most of the fire's been put out already."

I'm not entirely sure where these extra couple of hours a day are going to come from—I need to either

---

Gynaecologists—a necessary hurdle to proceed up the ranks. The exam is in two equally brutal parts and feels rather like the Labors of Hercules in that you're forced to do it to demonstrate your extraordinary dedication to the field more than anything else.

give up my frivolous hobby of sleeping or cut out my commute by living in a storage closet at work. Oh, and my exam's in four months, not six.

Monday, December 25, 2006

I don't particularly mind working Christmas Day— there are snacks everywhere, people on the whole are in a good mood, and there are very few worried well.*

Generally, people don't show up at the hospital on Christmas Day unless they're genuinely sick, genuinely in labor, or genuinely hate their families. (In which case, we've at least got some common ground.) I'm not convinced H sees it this way, as we exchange gifts at breakneck speed before seven a.m.

Tradition at St. Agatha's dictates that the on-call consultant† turns up and does ward rounds on Christmas Day, which eases the workload for the juniors. The consultant will also bring a bag of presents for the patients—toiletries, fruitcake, that sort of thing— because, well, it's pretty rotten being a hospital patient over Christmas, and the little things do make a differ-

---

* A lot of individuals (I'm not calling them patients; there's nothing wrong with them) come to the hospital under the misapprehension that they're in some way ill; they're known as the worried well. If this is because of something they've read online, they're called cyberchondriacs.

† Consultants are generally on call from home outside of normal working hours, giving telephone advice when needed and coming in only for major emergencies.

ence. Best of all, tradition has it that this consultant will be dressed as Santa Claus to do the rounds.

The nursing staff's disappointment is palpable when today's consultant, Dr. Hopkirk, turns up around ten a.m. wearing chinos and a sweater. Before the cries of "Grinch!" and "Ebenezer!" get too deafening, he explains that the last time he was on call on Christmas Day, he put on the outfit and beard for rounds and was halfway through when an elderly patient suddenly went into cardiac arrest. He dashed over and started CPR while a nurse went to fetch the crash cart. Unusually, the CPR was successful,* and the patient gasped back to life to the sight of a six-foot Santa lip-locked with her, his arms on her chest. "I can still hear her scream," he says.

"Go on," says one of the nurses, sounding like a child failing to hide her distress that her Christmas present is a calligraphy set and not a kitten. "Maybe just the hat?"

---

* If your heart stops, you're probably going to die. God is fairly strict on that matter. If you collapse on the street and a bystander starts cardiopulmonary resuscitation (CPR), then your chance of survival is around 8 percent. In hospital, with trained personnel, drugs, and defibrillators, it's only about twice that. People don't realize quite how horrific resuscitation is—undignified, brutal, and with a fairly woeful success rate. When discussing Do Not Resuscitate orders, relatives often want "everything to be done" without truly knowing what that means. Really, the form should say, "If your mother's heart stops, would you like us to break all her ribs and electrocute her?"

Wednesday, January 17, 2007

"In order to encourage use of public transport" there is no staff car park at the hospital—an admirable sentiment that would land me with a two-hour-and-twenty-minute commute each way. Instead, I've opted for a seventy-minute drive, leaving my wheels in the visitors' car park. The pricing system must have been dreamed up by people who realized the chances of winning the lottery more than once were pretty skeletal and thought there must be another way to raise a similar annual revenue. It's three pounds per hour with no discount for long stays and is applicable every hour of every day and every night except for Christmas, which presumably they decided would be greedy.

The only exception is for a woman in labor; she gets a parking voucher valid for three days when signed by the labor-ward supervisor. I'm on good terms with the supervisors—not so much for the fact that day in, day out I resolve obstetric emergencies but because I occasionally bring in a box of Krispy Kremes. As a result, they're happy to sign a parking voucher for me every few days and have therefore provided me with a *marché-gris* parking space for the past few months.

Today, however, the jig is up; my car has a clamp and a notice citing the hundred-and-twenty-pound fine for its removal jammed under the windshield wiper. I consider buying an angle grinder for fifty quid, but I've been at work twelve hours and just want to get to bed as quickly as possible. I grab the notice to find out who to call. The parking attendant has scrawled on the back, *Long fucking labor, pal.*

Sunday, January 21, 2007

Just when I was thinking it had been a while since the last episode of *Unexpected Objects Stuck in Orifices*, today a patient in her twenties presents to the ER unable to retrieve a bottle she'd put up there. Speculum* in—so what's it going to be this time? Chanel No. 5? Two liters of Dr Pepper? The magic potion I need to drink to take me to the next level of that Dungeons and Dragons game I abandoned twenty-four years ago? As it transpires, it's a medical sample bottle filled to the top with urine.

I can't work out the backstory, so I ask her to enlighten me. It turns out she has to provide her probation officer with clean urine samples, and so, rather than choosing the simpler option of not taking drugs, she has her mother piss in a jar that she then smuggles in vaginally and decants into the sample cup she's given by the probation officer. I think about the enormous volume of paperwork I'll generate for myself if I

---

* The *speculum* is a great clanking duckbill of a device used for looking inside the vagina. The first speculum was invented by an American surgeon called Sims back in 1845. He later wrote in his autobiography, "If there was anything I hated, it was investigating the organs of the female pelvis," which goes some way to explain why he devised such a hideous instrument.

document this in the notes, so I pretend I never asked the question and send her home.

Monday, January 29, 2007

My favorite patient died a couple of weeks ago, and it rather knocked the stuffing out of me. It was far from unexpected; KL was eighty in the shade with metastatic ovarian cancer, and she'd been on the ward as long as I'd worked on this unit, minus a couple of short-lived discharges home. Five foot nothing of Polish sass, with bright, twinkling eyes, she loved to tell long, meandering stories from back home that she would invariably get bored with the moment they got interesting—almost all of them ended with "Blah-blah-blah" and a vague wave of the hand.

Best of all, she despised my consultant, Professor Fletcher. She called him "old man" every time she saw him even though she had a good fifteen years on him, regularly prodded her finger into his chest when making a point, and once asked to see his line manager. I'd genuinely look forward to her stop on ward rounds—we'd always have a good chat and I really felt like I'd got to know her.

She immediately clocked I was Polish, despite three generations of my family living in England, breeding with Brits, and sending their offspring to expensive schools. She asked my original family name—I told her it was Strykowski. She thought it was sad that a good Polish name like that was out of commission, told me I should be proud of my heritage and change it back.

Over the months I'd met all of her children as well as numerous friends and neighbors who came to visit. "*Now* they like me!" she would say. Despite the joke, you could see why everyone did like her; she had a magnetic personality.

I was really upset when I heard she'd died. I decided I should go to the funeral—it felt like the right thing to do. I swapped out of clinic that afternoon so I could make it and let Professor Fletcher know I'd be attending, as a courtesy.

He told me I couldn't—doctors don't go to their patients' funerals, it's unprofessional, he said. I didn't quite understand why. His argument hinged on drawing a personal and professional line, which I agree with to an extent, but his tone seemed to suggest I was going along in order to seduce her grandchildren or get myself written into the will. I suspect that underpinning it is actually an old-fashioned sense that doctors have "lost" or "failed" if a patient dies; there's an element of blame or shame. Not really a sustainable attitude in gynaeoncology, where there's always going to be quite a high patient turnover. I was disappointed—partly because I'd had a suit dry-cleaned specially—but he's my boss and those were his very clear instructions.

Of course, I went to the funeral all the same, not

least because that's exactly the kind of fuck-you she'd have wanted to give him. It was a beautiful service, and I'm certain it was the right thing to do—for me and for the friends and family I'd met on the ward. Plus I was able to sleep with one of her grandchildren.*

---

* "I think you should point out that this is a joke," recommended one of the lawyers.

4

Senior House Officer—Post Three

I realize people everywhere moan about their salaries and think they deserve more, but I'm happy to look back on my time as an SHO with a bit of objectivity and declare I was profoundly underpaid. The money is utterly out of step with the level of responsibility you have—literally life-and-death decisions—plus there's the fact you've been to medical school for six years, worked as a doctor for three, and started to accrue postgraduate qualifications. Even if you think it's appropriate that you take home less money per week than a train driver, there's still the issue that each working week can involve over a hundred hours of unremitting slog, meaning the parking meters outside the hospital get a better hourly rate.

Doctors tend not to complain about the money, though. It's not a profession you go into to satisfy the dollar signs behind your eyes, whatever the occasional dead-mouthed politician may claim. Besides, even if you're unhappy with your salary, there's sod all you can do about it. It's all determined centrally and rolled out across the entire profession. Perhaps it's unhelpful to describe it as a salary; the NHS should call what they pay doctors a "stipend," acknowledging it's below the prevailing rate but that physicians are in the job because it's their calling rather than for any financial imperative.[*]

Nothing about the job plays along with the conventional reward structure for employees. There's no opportunity for a bonus—the closest that exists is "ash cash," where juniors get forty pounds a pop for signing a form for funeral directors confirming the patient about to be cremated doesn't have a pacemaker. (Pacemakers explode during the process, taking with them entire crematoria and congregations, as one family presumably found out during a particularly stressful funeral.) Thinking about it, that's pretty much the opposite of performance-related pay. There's no dazzling your superiors and leapfrogging over your peers or any opportunity for promotion; you progress up the ranks at a regulation rate.

Everyone seems to think doctors get upgraded on planes, but the only way that happens in reality is if the doctor puts on a suit—and then applies for a job

---

[*] Like the way priests get a stipend for their duty to God (or love of choirboys, depending on denomination).

in the city, earns more money, and buys a business-class ticket. I suppose you do have unlimited access to the informal medical opinions of every specialty if you begin to malfunction in any way. This is good, but it's just as well, as there's little chance you'd get the time off work to go to an outpatient clinic. But I'm not sure it's worth the flip side of providing medical advice to every friend at every opportunity. You'll hear "Could you just take a quick look?" more than you'll ever hear "Hey, it's great to see you."* My only small consolation was not having to give medical advice to relatives, what with most of my relatives being doctors.

All physicians come to grips with the lack of promotion and financial incentives, but it's harder to accept the fact that it's rare to get a "well done." The butlers at Buckingham Palace, who are under orders to float out of rooms backward and never make eye contact with the Queen, probably get more recognition. It didn't strike me for years, not until the fifth or sixth time I'd had my knuckles rapped for some trivial fuckup when a degree of human error had kicked in, that none of my consultants had ever taken me aside to say I was doing a good job or that I'd made a smart management decision, saved a life, cleverly thought on my feet, or stayed at work late for the thirtieth consecutive shift without complaining. Nobody joins the NHS looking for plaudits or expecting a gold star or a

---

* Tediously, this has morphed into something even worse now that I'm a TV writer. I'd take "What do you think about this rash?" over "What do you think about this script?" any day.

cookie every time they do a good job, but you'd think it might be basic psychology (and common sense) to occasionally acknowledge, if not reward, good behavior to get the most out of your staff.

Patients tended to get it, though. When one of them said thank you, you knew they meant it—even if it felt like it wasn't for anything special, just one of the smaller horrors thrown at you that day. I've kept every single card a patient has given me. Birthday and Christmas cards from family and friends would always get thrown away, but these guys survived every house move, escaping even my cathartic clear-out of medical paperwork once it was all over. They were little fist bumps that kept me going, rays of thoughtfulness from my patients that hit the spot when bosses couldn't, or wouldn't, oblige.

It took until now, my third job as an SHO, to feel properly recognized by a consultant for the first time. A few months into my contract, my clinical supervisor said that a registrar was leaving the post early for a research job and asked if I'd be interested in a temporary promotion. She told me she'd been very impressed with my work in the department. I knew this was a lie; she'd met me twice—once at induction and once to bollock me for starting a patient on oral rather than intravenous antibiotics. She'd clearly just looked through all the résumés and clocked that I had worked as an SHO for the longest. But sometimes it doesn't matter how they spot you as long as they actually *do*, so I beamed and said I'd be delighted.

I also realized this could make a significant practical difference to me. Three years into our relationship, H and I were taking the next step into adulthood and looking to buy a flat. I'd decided to sacrifice a shorter commute so we could have a permanent base, a place to actually call home, somewhere you can hang a picture on the wall without being docked fifty quid from your rental deposit. Most nonmedical friends were clambering onto the second rung of the property ladder by then, and you know what it's like when your friends are all doing something and you're not. Whether it's fingering someone at a party, taking your driving test, or dropping hundreds of thousands of pounds on a dungeon with dry rot—nobody wants to be left behind.

Because every penny of salary helps with getting a mortgage, I asked the consultant if I'd be paid more while I was the acting registrar. She laughed so long and so hard I'm pretty sure you could hear it through two sets of double doors over on the labor ward.

Monday, February 12, 2007

Prescribing a morning-after pill in the ER. The patient says, "I slept with three guys last night. Will one pill be enough?"

Thursday, February 22, 2007

Spent the morning going through three months of bank statements with the mortgage broker so he can assess my expenditures. "You don't . . . go out much, do you?" he says, totting it up. For once I'm grateful for my job—we wouldn't have saved up enough for a deposit if I were allowed the normal social life of someone in his late twenties.

It's reasonably depressing looking at where the money goes: a lot of coffee, a lot of petrol, a lot of takeaway pizza—necessities and practicalities. Not much in the way of fun or extracurricular frippery—no pubs, restaurants, cinemas, or holidays. Hang on, what's that? There we go—theater tickets! Shortly followed by a payment to a florist after I'd bailed on H at the last minute. Depressingly, it happened frequently enough that I couldn't even remember the particular emergency or staffing crisis on that occasion.

Wednesday, February 28, 2007

In gynae clinic, I go online to look up some management guidelines for a patient. The trust's IT department has blocked the Royal College of Obstetrics and Gynaecology website and classified it as pornography.

Monday, March 12, 2007

Pretty sure that if obs and gynae goes arse over tit I could retrain in psychiatry in about fifteen minutes—I've basically taught myself how to do it over the course of a dozen conversations with Simon. Tonight I was pretty stressed when he called and had a bit of a moan about work. Unexpectedly, this really seemed to help him. Either he's a horrible sadist and likes the idea of me having an awful day or it's comforting for him to know that everyone else has shit going on in their lives too. Misery loves company, after all—you only have to look in the doctors' mess to know that.

Maybe it's like when you're in a proper relationship for the first time and you meet the family and you see it's not just *your* family that's a miserable fucked-up mess with dozens of dark secrets and grotesque dinner-table habits. I finished today's call with Simon in hysterics after I told him a lump of placenta flew into my mouth during a manual removal and I had to go to occupational health about it. He may well be a sadist, come to think of it.

Thursday, March 15, 2007

I ask a patient in prenatal clinic how many weeks she is now. There's a long pause. Cogs turn. A camera slowly pans across a wasteland. Math isn't everyone's strong point, but I'm after the number between six and forty that people must constantly ask her about. Finally:

"In total?"

Yes, in total.

"God, I couldn't even tell you in months . . ."

Has she got amnesia? Is she a clone of another woman currently being held prisoner in an evil sci-fi villain's lair? I start to ask when her last period was, and she interrupts.

"Well, I'm thirty-two in June, so that's got to be more than a thousand weeks . . ."

Christ.

Thursday, March 22, 2007

Idea for *Shark Tank*: a bleeper with a snooze button.

Thursday, April 5, 2007

Revenge is a dish best served cold—so long as it doesn't end up poisoning the wrong person. I was called to assess a patient on the ward; she'd had a laparoscopic drainage of a pelvic abscess in the morning and her pulse had been raised all evening. According to the notes, this lady was in her midfifties and had discovered on her wedding anniversary that she wasn't the only person to have received a pearl necklace from her husband. Her reaction was seemingly straight out of niche porn—she took herself and her husband's credit card off to Trinidad and Tobago and had sex with as many men as she could over the course of a fortnight, expanding her bedroom (and beach) repertoire to include anal sex.

Back home, bowlegged but unbowed, she was soon having terrible abdominal pain, plus producing purulent monsoons from both her Trinidad *and* her Tobago. She was diagnosed with pelvic inflammatory disease,* and even IV antibiotics couldn't persuade it to sod off—seemingly, there's some pretty weapons-grade gonorrhea going round the Caribbean. Today's procedure would hopefully get her back on the road.

It turned out her raised pulse wasn't due to any surgical complications but because she was in floods of tears. I asked what was up and she told me her eighteen-year-old son was coming over tomorrow to visit, and she didn't know what to say to him—how would he react when he found out why she was in the hospital? I assured her that an eighteen-year-old boy would rather peel his testicles and douse them in malt vinegar than ask any questions at all about why his mother is on a gynecology ward. The phrase

---

* *Pelvic inflammatory disease*, or PID, is when untreated gonorrhea or chlamydia spreads north and gunks up the pelvic organs—it can be tricky to treat and even result in permanent pelvic pain. It's also one of the main causes of female infertility. Basically, use condoms or you might end up not needing them at all.

women's problems alone—especially if delivered in hushed tones while staring straight into his eyes— would have him changing the subject immediately, even if he had to start a small fire as a distraction. Tears over and pulse back down to normal. Although she might want to think up a plausible excuse for that incredible suntan . . .

Monday, April 9, 2007

Results out today. I have somehow passed my MRCOG part one exam and am celebrating in the pub with Ron. Unfortunately, drinks are strictly nonalcoholic as I have to head straight off afterward to a night shift, and I gather turning up drunk is frowned upon. Ron recently got through his postgraduate accountancy exams, so we compare notes. While his firm cut down his hours so he could study, I had to squeeze in as much studying as my bloodshot eyes would allow after work. Ron had a full month of study leave before the exam; I applied for a week off, but gaps in the schedule meant that it ended up getting canceled at the last minute, without discussion. His firm paid for all exam fees and materials; I had to shell out three hundred pounds for textbooks, five hundred for a course, a hundred for online learning resources, and four hundred for the exam itself, a grand total of thirteen hundred pounds—a mere two-thirds of my monthly take-home pay.

My carefully considered exam answers didn't even get seen by a human—it's a multiple-choice test and you fill in the answers in pencil on a grid, which then gets scanned and marked by a computer. I show Ron the RCOG pencil I pinched.

He immediately gets a promotion and a pay raise for passing his exam; all mine means is that I'm now eligible to take the second part of the exam.

"No. All it means," says Ron sympathetically, "is that you spent thirteen hundred pounds on a pencil."

Thursday, April 19, 2007

An e-mail from Infection Control informs all doctors that long-sleeved shirts are now banned in clinical environments. Some researchers swabbed a bunch of cuffs and discovered it would be more hygienic for us to wear shirts made out of fresh human feces and poorly sealed vials of Ebola. The same apparently applies to neckties, which dangle down, bobbing in and out of various festering wounds and cross-pollinating bugs across the hospital like polyester honeybees with a death wish.

We are henceforth instructed to wear short-sleeved shirts, so I brush aside any hope of making the cover of *Vogue* while at work and go shopping to invest my savings in five of the things. These short-sleeved numbers, we are told, may be worn either with no tie or with a bow tie—giving us the option of dressing like an airline steward or a pedophile. I'll go without, thanks. Tea? Coffee? Hot towel?

Wednesday, May 2, 2007

I finish explaining the risks of a cesarean section to a couple. "Any questions at all?" I ask the room.

"Yes," chimes in their six-year-old. "Do you think Jesus was black?"

Saturday, May 5, 2007

In lieu of an incentive scheme at work, I've invented my own perks: I take scrubs home for pajamas and steal the odd patient meal at night. It's one a.m., I'm absolutely starving, and this is my only chance for some food for the next seven hours, so I sidle into the gynae-ward kitchen. Clearly I'm not the only one with an eye for a freebie; there's a new sign up on the fridge warning staff that meals are strictly for patients only. As security systems go, it's not exactly sophisticated—they'll struggle to prevent the more determined thief with printer paper, Scotch tape, and Comic Sans alone.

Tonight's delicacy is "Savory Mycoprotein Mince with Sultanas." It's like they hired an agency to come up with the least appealing menu options possible. I think I'll just take my chances and let nervous energy and Red Bull keep me going.

Saturday, May 12, 2007

My philosophy on flights is to get so hammered that no right-minded airline steward would want me anywhere near a sick passenger, which has served me well these past few years.* Karma repaid me tonight, not on the flight itself but twelve hours later. I was in Glasgow for the weekend and going back to the hotel after dinner and drinks and drinks and drinkssssssss with Ron and his wife, Hannah.

Walking down Bath Street at one a.m., we see three guys in their late teens hanging around some basement steps outside a shop door surrounded by an extraordinary amount of blood. It looked unreal, like a murder scene on a low-budget, late-night drama. They were all the worse for wear—though probably no worse than any of us—and one was exsanguinating from what looked like a big arterial bleed on his forearm. Impossible to guess how much blood was sprayed and pooled around, but it couldn't have been less than a liter. He was conscious, though barely, and nothing was being done to stem the blood loss.

---

* My family are much nicer people than me. One Christmas, British Airways sent my dad a pair of round-trip tickets to anywhere in the world as a thank-you for answering the "Is there a doctor on board?" call and handing out some antihistamines from the medicine box. My brother (also a GP) was unimpressed—he'd spent the entire duration of a budget airline flight managing an urgent cardiac situation with extremely limited resources and didn't even get the words "Thank you" as a thank-you, let alone a free trip to Bali.

I sobered up extremely quickly and told them I was a doctor. The friends were pointing at the smashed glass door and repeatedly telling me he'd tripped and fallen, as if the fact he'd clearly broken into a newsstand was anyone's main concern here. They'd called an ambulance already, but I had Ron phone 999 to expedite its appearance and asked Hannah to rip up T-shirts to make tourniquets. I held the guy's arm up high and squeezed hard. His pulse was slow and thready,[*] and he was drifting in and out of consciousness. I kept talking, talking, talking—telling him the ambulance was really close, that I was a doctor, that everything was going to be fine. It doesn't matter how many times you say it or whether any of it is true— well, at least the "doctor" part is true—you have to believe it, because *they* need to believe it.

It felt like he was on the brink of cardiac arrest and I was going through the steps of CPR in my head so I wouldn't need to think twice when he did. Was this even legal—drunk in charge of an emergency? I was confident I was managing the situation correctly, but it wouldn't look *great* if he died with me in this state. Mercifully, the ambulance arrived almost immediately and they whisked him away, filling him with the fluids he needed to save his life. All's well that ends well,

---

[*] If you lose blood, then your pulse usually speeds up—your heart needs to work extra hard to get oxygen around the body, given there's less blood to transport it. When the pulse becomes slow in this situation, it generally means the body is getting exhausted and preparing to throw in the towel.

but I had a terrible feeling of impotence waiting for the ambulance to pull up. Back in the hotel I poured myself a £12 miniature from the minibar and realized that even on a plane, I'd have had more resources to help him. The whiskey would have been cheaper too.

Monday, May 14, 2007

In the doctors' mess, my friend Zac—currently working in orthopedics—tells me that he always muddles the words *shoulder* and *elbow* in his mind and has to really concentrate before using either term. Before I even have time to process this and what it could mean for his next patient, an intensive care registrar chimes in from the next sofa: Since childhood, she's always malapropped the words *coma* and *cocoon*. The more she tries to remember which is which, the more her mind convinces her she's got it the wrong way round. She shows us a piece of paper in her wallet that reads,

Cocoon = Insect. Coma = Patient.

This, we hear, helps prevent the admittedly hilarious scenario of sitting down an inconsolable spouse to break the news that her husband is in a cocoon.

Tuesday, June 12, 2007

It's five minutes until my shift ends and I need to get away in time to go out for dinner. Naturally, I'm asked to assess a patient. She's got a second-degree tear,* and the midwife looking after her tells me she hasn't been signed off to repair those yet.†

> Me: I haven't been signed off to do them either.
> Midwife: You don't need to get signed off to do things—you're a doctor. [Depressing but true.]
> Me: Isn't there another midwife who can do it?
> Midwife: She's on her break.
> Me: I'm on my break. [Untrue.]
> Midwife: You don't get breaks. [Depressing but true.]
> Me (*pleading, in a tone of voice I've never managed before, like I've unlocked a secret level*

---

* Having a baby can rip your undercarriage to shreds, there's no getting around it, especially if you're a first-time mum. Trojan should take its cue from cigarette manufacturers and show photos of postpartum perinea on its packaging—no woman would look at that and want to risk getting pregnant. A first-degree tear goes through the skin, a second-degree tear goes into the perineal muscles, a third-degree tear involves the anal sphincter, and a fourth-degree tear rips your leg off or something.

† Doctors' and midwives' roles are fairly well defined in most aspects of the labor ward—midwives are responsible for normal deliveries; doctors are involved when there are worries about mum's or baby's well-being or the progress of labor. Who gets the sewing kit out for first- and second-degree tears is a grayer area than your granny's vagina.

of my vocal cords): But it's my *birthday*. [Depressing but true.]

Midwife: It's a labor ward—it's always someone's birthday.

Tuesday, June 19, 2007

An e-mail to all clinical staff to let us know that a psychiatric patient has been transferred to the respiratory ward following a diagnosis of pneumonia. But this wasn't the kind of "Say hello if you see him" notice you'd get if a new kid transferred to your school. Yesterday it was discovered he'd been wandering around the ward minesweeping like the last aunt at a wedding, downing the contents of every sputum cup he found on fellow patients' bedside tables.

We are advised to send all clinical samples *immediately* to the lab and not to leave any in easy reach for the time being. Someone has replied-all with *Yuck*, which feels rather like watching a nuclear reactor explode and saying, *Oh, dear.*

Tuesday, June 26, 2007

I've been in the doghouse for days now. We were at H's friend Luna's house; Luna is pregnant, and just before dinner she whipped out a photo album of their recent 3-D scans. I suspected that my thoughts on 3-D scans—that they serve no purpose other than keeping 3-D-scanning companies rich and boring the anuses off dinner-party guests—would go down like a cup of cold sick, so I had a polite flick through along with everyone else.

"Everything seem okay?" Luna asked me. I wanted to say, *Looks the same as they all fucking do*, but I figured that might lose the room, so I just smiled sweetly, handed the photos back, and said, "She looks perfect." The temperature in the room dropped about ten degrees and murder flashed discernibly across Luna's eyes. "She? *She?*"

It's the first time I've dropped the ball on this, so to speak, and worst of all, it was with a friend, not a patient. Dinner felt like it took a fortnight; eye contact avoided, plates plomped unceremoniously in front of me.

It didn't help that tensions were already running high at home. Two weeks ago, our flat purchase fell through. It seems that, with a total disregard for my blood pressure and a relationship slightly fraying at the edges, the owners decided not to sell it after all. I rather suspected they'd merely decided not to sell it to *us*, probably because someone else had offered them a bit more money. Luckily, we've only spent a couple of thousand fucking pounds on solicitors and surveys and whatnot. I know more about this flat—that I will now never set foot in again—than I do about any of my closest blood relations. Everyone tells us that these things happen for a reason. In our case, the reason is that the world favors bastards and clearly wants us to spend our every spare moment with real estate agents for the next few months.

But life goes on, even if it's peppered with annoying reminders of the lost flat. The depleted bank account, for one, and the fact that, unless I take a five-minute PTSD-avoiding detour, I drive past the flat that got away every morning on my journey to work. And today—amazingly, just to prove there's no escape—the couple who screwed us over turned up in prenatal clinic. I'd not met them before, but there was their address in front of me, the exact same address that's permanently scarring my happiness.

In a Tarantino movie, this would be the part where I produce two samurai swords and unleash a ten-minute tirade about honor, vengeance, and respect, then decapitate them. In reality I just said, "Hi, I'm Adam, one of the doctors," and they had no idea. Issues of morality, probity, and legality sadly restrict revenge opportunities to near enough zero, so I conducted their appointment to the best of my abilities, albeit through gritted teeth. I wasn't 100 percent sure that the baby was cephalic,* so I quickly ran the scanner over the mother. Baby was the right way up and all was well. "Do you want to see the heart beating?" I asked them.

---

* *Cephalic* means baby is head down—this is normal. The opposite is breech, meaning bum-first. Breech presentation occurs in 3 percent of pregnancies, and famous examples include Emperor Nero, Kaiser Wilhelm, Frank Sinatra, and Billy Joel. If you win a pub quiz off this, you owe me a pint.

"There it is—all looks normal there. There's an arm, another arm, that's a leg, that's his penis . . . Oh, didn't you know?"

Saturday, June 30, 2007

There's a news story in the paper about a hospital orderly who's been jailed for pretending to be a doctor for the last few years. Just finished one of those shifts where I wondered if I could get away with pretending to be an orderly.

Tuesday, July 10, 2007

I clearly need to change my patter. It usually goes something like "I couldn't see anything on the ultrasound just by looking with a probe on the tummy—doesn't mean there's anything to worry about, early pregnancies can often be very difficult to see this way. Would it be okay if I did an ultrasound using an internal probe to get a better view?" But after today's incident, should my license to practice remain intact, my new spiel will be "I couldn't see anything on the ultrasound just by looking with a probe on the tummy—doesn't mean there's anything to worry about, early pregnancies can often be very difficult to see this way. Would it be okay if I did an ultrasound using an internal probe to get a better view? In a few seconds' time I'm going to rummage in a drawer and pull out a condom and a tube of K-Y Jelly. Just to be clear—the condom is a cover for the ultrasound probe and the K-Y Jelly is to lubricate it. When you see what's in my hands, please do not scream so loudly that three members of the staff come rushing into the room."

Monday, July 23, 2007

Sending a patient home from the day-surgery unit following laparoscopic sterilization. I tell her she can have sex again as soon as she feels ready but to use alternative contraception until her next period. I nod at her husband and say, "That means *he* has to wear a condom." I can't quite work out why their faces are a picture of horror, melting like the Nazis at the end of *Raiders of the Lost Ark*. What have I said? It's perfectly good advice, right? I look at them both again and realize the man is actually her father.

Tuesday, July 31, 2007

One of the house officers turned up in the ER last night, having attempted suicide with an overdose of antidepressants. There's a shared sense of numbness amongst the doctors. The only surprise is that it doesn't happen more often—you're given huge responsibility, minimal supervision, and absolutely no pastoral support.* You work yourself to exhaustion, pushing yourself beyond what could be reasonably expected of you, and end up constantly feeling like you don't know what you're do-ing. Sometimes it just feels that way, and you're actu-ally doing fine—and sometimes you *really* don't know what you're doing.

Happily, this occasion is the latter; the house officer didn't know what she was doing and took a completely harmless dose of antidepressants. In any other profes-sion, if someone's job drove her to attempt suicide, you'd expect some kind of inquiry into what happened and a concerted effort to make sure it never happened again. Yet nobody said anything—we all just heard from friends, like we were in the school playground. I doubt we'd have got so much as an e-mail if she'd died. I'm pretty unshockable, but I'll never cease to be amazed by hospitals' willful ineptitude when it comes to caring for their own staff.

---

* A 2015 study by the Medical Protection Society showed that 85 percent of doctors have experienced mental-health issues and 13 percent admitted to suicidal feelings. A 2009 paper in the *British Journal of Psychiatry* showed that young female doctors in the UK are two and a half times more likely than other women to kill themselves.

5

Registrar—Post One

As a house officer, you think your registrar (I'll save you turning back to the comparison chart: registrar = fellow) is unimpeachably correct and clever, like God maybe, or Google, and you try not to bother them under almost any circumstance. The SHO is your port of call whenever you get stuck and need an answer, the safety net of some wise words just a quick bleep away. And then, before you know it, the registrar is *you*.

In obs and gynae, it means you'll frequently be the most senior person in clinic. You'll lead the ward rounds more often than not. You're expected to teach medical students. You're expected to perform all but the meatiest of operations. Most crucially, you run the labor ward. There are senior registrars and potentially even consultants available if you hit DEFCON 1, but this is the grade where you're generally responsible for keeping a dozen laboring mums and babies alive. This one probably needs a cesarean, these two are going to need an instrumental delivery, this one's hemorrhaging. You become amazing at prioritizing. It's like you're living in a constant logic puzzle, the one with the boat, the fox, the chicken, and the bag of grain. Except there are a dozen chickens, they're all delivering triplets, and the boat's made of sugar.

It sounds horrific—and at times it was—but the day I started as a registrar, I had a huge spring in my step. Not since I'd graduated from medical school had I felt so optimistic—I was practically shitting confetti. I was suddenly halfway to becoming a consultant, enjoying the Wednesday afternoon of my metaphorical week. Not only was a senior job just a few years away, I could actually picture myself doing it, maybe even doing it well. It felt like everything at work and home was clicking into place, like I'd finally figured out I'd been holding the map upside down all this time. For once my life didn't seem that depressing compared to nonmedical friends. I had a flat, a new(er) car, and a (more or less) stable relationship. I felt satisfied. Not smug or complacent, but just in marked contrast to the years I'd felt somehow *unsatisfied* with the way things had been going.

I realized that most of my colleagues weren't so lucky, especially when it came to their home lives. Mine was largely held together by superhuman levels of tolerance and understanding; most doctors' relationships crumbled after a year or so. The cracks that they all develop would appear far too early, like some bizarre premature-aging disorder.

Certainly the hours don't help. After four or five years of intravenous NHS Kool-Aid, staying late, arriving early, and filling in for colleagues have become fully formed habits. A widely held belief among nondoctors is that there's some degree of choice involved in coming home at ten p.m. rather than eight. But really, the only choice is whether you fuck over yourself or your patients. The former is annoying, the latter means that people die—so it's not really a choice at all. The system runs on a skeleton staff and, on all but the quietest shifts, relies on the charity of doctors staying beyond their contracted hours to get things done. It would be against everything you stand for to knowingly compromise patient safety, so you don't—which means you stay late after almost every shift. Of course, doctors aren't alone in working late—you could say the same of lawyers and bankers, but at least they can become "weekend warriors," letting down their hair and their ancestors in a forty-eight-hour blast of unremitting hedonism. Doctors' weekends are usually spent at work.

But it's more than just the hours; you're generally no fun to be around when you get home. You're exhausted, you're snappy from a stressful day, and you even manage to deny your partners the normal post-work chat of bitching about their colleagues. They know as soon as they start on their workplace quibbles—which presumably don't involve any near-death experiences unless they're tightrope walkers, firefighters, or counter staff at a drive-thru Burger King—you'll reflexively talk about the horrors of your own day.

Your subconscious ends up making a decision on your behalf. Either you fail to tune out the bad stuff from work and become permanently distracted and haunted at home or you develop a hardened emotional exoskeleton, which apparently isn't considered an ideal quality in a partner.

A few of my colleagues had kids by this point and lived their lives in constant childcare hell, adding "guilt" to the psychology textbook of emotions that a career in medicine bestows on you. I don't have kids, but I could understand what a gut-wrench it was for my colleagues to settle for a good-night phone call with their children rather than tucking them in and reading them *The Gruffalo*. Or, more often than not, they'd miss the call altogether because the labor ward was in meltdown. A friend who worked in general surgery once couldn't go to his own son's emergency surgery because he was performing nonemergency surgery on someone else's son and no one could cover for him.

Once I became a registrar, I noticed an interesting paradox: while you become an expert in prioritizing at work, you generally become even worse at prioritizing in real life. But for a while there, I felt like the exception who proved the rule—the one guy who had his shit together in some small way, plates all spinning away nicely. Now I just had to make sure none of them smashed . . .

Thursday, August 16, 2007

A horror story. Patient GL, whose genetic makeup appears to be 50 percent goji-berry recipes and 50 percent yoga mats, has announced she wants to eat her placenta. The midwife and I both pretend not to hear this—first because we don't know what the hospital protocol is, and second because it's completely revolting. GL calls it *placentophagia* to make it sound more official, which doesn't particularly wash; you can make anything sound official by translating it into ancient Greek.*

She explains how natural it is among other mammals, which is another somewhat defective argument—we don't let other mammals do things like run for Parliament or drive buses, nor do we normalize other things they do like fucking the furniture or eating their young (or *pedophagia*, as she'd presumably call it).

I turn the conversation to the more pressing matter of clapping some forceps on her baby's head and getting it out. This happens smoothly and the baby is fine—and will continue to be until it gets homeschooled and taken on all-naked, yurt-based family

---

* *Cholelithoproctophilia* would be shoving gallstones up your arse, but I've just made it up. *Orbitobelonephilia*—sticking needles in your eyes. *Craniophallic anastomosis*—dickhead.

holidays. A couple of minutes later, I'm delivering the placenta and look up to have the awkward discussion about what GL would like me to do with it. She has a kidney dish in her hands and is shoveling handfuls of blood clots into her mouth.

"Isn't *this* the placenta?" she asks, blood dribbling out of the corner of her mouth like she's the disgusting progeny of Dracula and the Cookie Monster. I explain that it's just some clots I left in a bowl after delivering the baby. She turns ashen, then green. Clearly blood isn't the delicious postdelivery snack she imagines placenta might be. She holds up the kidney dish and vomits into, onto, and around it. Sorry, I mean *experiences hematemesis.*

Tuesday, October 2, 2007

Retrieve my phone from the locker after an unremitting day on the labor ward. Seven missed calls from Simon and a bunch of voicemails, all from this morning. I hesitate before pressing Play—I know in my heart it'll be too late already; I'm already half preparing what to say to the coroner. Turns out Simon's pocket-dialed me, the little bastard.

Wednesday, October 24, 2007

It's a quiet night on the labor ward so I go to my on-call room, lie in bed, and piss around on Facebook for a bit. Someone has posted a link to a bucket-list quiz, where you tick off, from a checklist of a hundred items, various things you've achieved in your life. Have you visited the Great Wall of China? Ridden an ostrich? Been eaten out by one of Barry Manilow's security team in a Las Vegas infinity pool? It turns out I've done very few things at all. I check my e-mail, then have a wank.[*]

Mid-wank, the crash bleeper[†] goes off. Scrub trousers back on, I rush into a delivery room—the mother is pushing and there's an extremely worrying CTG. Within a minute of walking into the room, I have delivered the baby by forceps extraction. Mother and baby both fine, good old me. I can now write my own bucket list and tick off "Delivered a baby while still erect."

---

[*] I don't know what the GMC position is regarding wanking in on-call rooms. An e-mail to them asking for clarification sat unsent in my drafts folder for over a month when I was putting this book together until I chickened out and deleted it. But we've all done it. Basically, make sure your doctor uses the hand gel when he rushes into your room at night.

[†] For life-and-death emergencies, you can be summoned by a crash bleep—your bleeper is granted the power of speech and tells you exactly where to run to, saving valuable seconds.

Thursday, November 1, 2007

I've barely started an emergency cesarean when my SHO bursts into the operating theater to tell me that a patient in another room has a non-reassuring trace and might need an instrumental delivery. My senior registrar is performing some complicated and repulsive emergency gynae op in the main OR and this SHO is a GP trainee on a six-month placement, so it's my show entirely. I get her to take a photo of the CTG on her phone so I can see how bad it is and attempt to construct some sort of a plan.

By the time she pops back into the OR, I've delivered the baby and am starting to sew up the uterus. The trace is much worse than the SHO described, and I have another fifteen minutes of needlework still to go. I put in another stitch to stop the uterus bleeding and ask the scrub nurse to rest a large wet swab over the patient's open abdomen (leaving her looking like a horrendous Teletubby), then make my apologies and run off to perform a quick forceps delivery on the other baby. I've barely got the tongs off its head when the emergency buzzer blares from the room next door. Another nasty trace, this time needing a vacuum extraction, then management of a postpartum hemorrhage afterward for good measure.

By the time I get back to the OR to polish off my original cesarean, it's nearly ninety minutes later, and when *that* one's done, it's time to hand over to the morning registrar. I tell him my tale of superheroism, expecting him to suggest they rename the hospital after me. All I get in reply is a "Yeah, that happens," like I've mentioned the coffee shop has run out of *pains aux raisins*.

Monday, November 5, 2007

Patient in prenatal clinic told me she was taking Dorothy every morning because she was feeling stressed. Who's Dorothy? Some great-aunt she was escorting down to the shops as a strange kind of chill-out exercise, like a mental-health-assistance dog? She informed me Dorothy was the street name for ketamine.*

"Does it help with the stress?" I asked—and was genuinely interested in the answer.

Monday, November 12, 2007

All surgical staff have been summoned to a lecture on patient safety. Last week a patient had his completely healthy left kidney removed, leaving him with only a completely useless right kidney.

We're reminded that in the last three years, neurosurgeons in the UK have drilled holes in the wrong side of a patient's skull fifteen times. Fifteen times they

---

* Other terms for ketamine include *K*, *Kit Kat*, and *Special K*. Although if she'd told me she was having Special K every morning, I may well have missed the reference.

couldn't tell left from right while holding a Black and Decker to someone's cranium. Feels like grounds for retiring the "It's hardly brain surgery" maxim.

The hospital is very keen that mistakes like the great kidney snafu aren't repeated—although it's slightly too late for this poor guy, whose ashes have presumably just been scattered on the wrong beach.

The upshot is that new hospital protocol states any patient going to the OR must have a large arrow drawn in Sharpie pen on his left or right leg, as appropriate, to indicate the side being operated on. I put my hand up and ask what happens if the patient already has a tattoo of an arrow on the wrong leg. Decent laugh from the lecture hall and my consultant calls me a fucking clown.

Tuesday, November 13, 2007

I receive an e-mail from Dr. Vane, director of Clinical Governance, advising me that if a patient has a tattoo of an arrow on either leg, it should be covered up with Micropore tape and a new arrow drawn in Sharpie on the correct leg. This will now be included in the policy document, and he thanks me for my valuable contribution.

Tuesday, January 8, 2008

The population is getting fatter faster than a mobility scooter hurtling toward McDonald's at closing time. Today our labor-ward operating table is being replaced for the second time in as many years because last month a woman exceeded the weight capacity for the recently acquired "obese table."

I realize it's a complicated issue, but surely being so big that special equipment has to be ordered for you would be the first clue that now would be a good time to offload some timber.

The even newer table has enormous wings that flap up from the sides to prevent "overspill," like an industrial version of the dinner table that grandma can extend at Christmas to fit on all the extra vol-au-vents. I reckon you could comfortably rest a medium-size warship on it—it took ten men, some hydraulic equipment, and the best part of two hours to get it into the OR. I presume the next issue will be the table crashing through the floor one day mid-cesarean, killing the entire dermatology department beneath us.

Saturday, January 19, 2008

Today I tipped into full-blown Stockholm syndrome and decided to go into work on a Saturday off. "If you're having an affair, you can just tell me, you know," H said.

I'd performed my first TAH BSO* yesterday and wanted to check if the patient was doing okay. Every time my phone buzzed this morning, I'd assumed it was a message from the weekend team to tell me her wound had exploded or I'd punctured her bowel, severed a ureter, or let her quietly bleed to death internally. I basically just needed a bit of reassurance to stop myself going insane.

Obviously, when I got there I saw she was absolutely fine and had already been evaluated by my colleague Fred. I immediately felt bad—I'd hate him to think I didn't trust him to do his job properly (although I don't), so I nimbly hurried off the ward in order to escape unnoticed. Or not so nimbly—I bumped into him on my way out and had to pretend I was "just passing by" and thought I'd stop in to see if she was okay. "Don't blame you," Fred said, shrugging, and told me his first major op had died in hospital. He'd checked on her obsessively and planned her post-op care meticulously and then, on the day she was meant to go home, she'd choked to death on an egg and cress sandwich.

I'm now half considering making my patient nil-by-mouth until discharge, just to be on the safe side. Having "just passed by," I begin the hour-long drive back home and think about what H said earlier. Even if I

---

* *Total abdominal hysterectomy and bilateral salpingo-oophorectomy (TAH BSO)* is the removal of the uterus, cervix, tubes, and ovaries. Salpingo-oophorectomy has three o's in a row, which has to be some kind of record.

wanted to have an affair, I honestly think I'd be too tired to unzip my trousers.

Tuesday, February 26, 2008

About to perform a hysteroscopy* on patient FR, and as I'm talking through the procedure, she asks, "What's the worst that could happen?" Patients ask this all the time, and I wish they wouldn't because obviously the truthful answer is they could die. In her case, as with almost everyone who asks this, the chances of death are infinitesimal, but the question forces me to name-drop the Reaper immediately before the operation.

For the past few months, whenever someone has asked, "What's the worst that could happen?" I've replied, "The world could explode." This generally has the effect of making the patient realize she's catastrophizing and breaks the ice a little. Plus, it's not a lie— one day it will, and doubtless I'll be working on the labor ward when it does.

On this occasion, FR is a fervent believer that the world *is* going to end in the next five years and she

---

* Putting a camera inside the uterus. One of the mainstays of gynecology investigations, principally used for abnormal bleeding, but also a traditional procedure if you don't really know what else to do. It was first performed in 1869, and most units don't seem to have bought new equipment since.

invites me to a David Icke* lecture at Brixton Academy next week. I might even go. What's the worst that could happen?

Friday, February 29, 2008

Special occasions tend to call for patients to insert special types of objects into their vaginas and recta. Christmas in particular has rewarded me well, with a stuck fairy ("Do you want it back?" "Yeah, bit of a rinse and she'll be grand"), a grossly swollen vulva from a mistletoe contact allergy, and mild vaginal burns from a patient stuffing a string of lights inside and turning them on (bringing new meaning to the phrase "I put the Christmas lights up myself"). This is my first leap year working as a doctor and the Great British public have pulled it out of the bag for me with a very, very specific injury.

Patient JB decided to take advantage of tradition and propose to her boyfriend—going to the expense of buying an engagement ring, the trouble of putting it inside a Kinder Surprise egg, and the imagination of inserting it vaginally. She would suggest some finger work to her partner, he would discover it, retrieve it, and then she would go down on one knee (and, presumably, him). Equal parts unexpected, disgust-

---

* Icke is a professional conspiracy theorist and Holocaust denier who gives inexorably long, mad speeches.

ing, and, I suppose, romantic. Unfortunately, he was unable to retrieve it as planned—it had rotated itself lengthwise, and no amount of shoogling from either of them would get this particular goose to lay her golden egg. Remarkably, she was so keen to maintain the surprise she wouldn't tell him what she'd done or why, but eventually they decided this was a hospital matter, so we met in cubicle three. It was a very easy delivery with a pair of sponge-holding forceps.

She hadn't told me about the contents of the egg either at this point, so there was a moment of confusion for both me and the boyfriend when she asked him to open it. I gave him a pair of latex gloves, sandblasting the very last pico-trace of romance from the scenario. She popped the question and he said yes, presumably out of shock, or fear of what a woman who does that with a Kinder Surprise would do to him if spurned. I wonder where the best man will keep the wedding bands during the ceremony?

Monday, March 17, 2008

I'm unsure who decided that junior doctors have so much spare time on our hands that we should conduct annual clinical audits, but the audit meeting is this week, so I'm sitting reviewing patient notes after my night shift, going through the motions like Lady Chatterley in her marriage to the cockless Sir Clifford. As well as collecting my official audit data on APGAR scores* I have spotted an interesting incidental finding and have put together some data on that too.

Introduction

On our unit, 2,500 babies are delivered annually, of which roughly 750 are cesarean sections. The surgeon records hand-written operation notes for every patient, representing the permanent legal record of the procedure.

Methods

I personally reviewed the operative notes of 382 cesarean sections, representing all such procedures performed between January and June 2007.

Results

In 109 cases (28.5 percent) the surgeon performing the procedure has misspelled *cesarean* as *cesarian*.

---

*   *APGAR scores* are the standard measure of how well a newborn baby is doing—they get marked on Appearance, Pulse, Grimace, Activity, and Respiration. It was devised by a doctor called Virginia Apgar, which makes me think she chose arbitrary measures just because they fitted with her surname. Like if I decided that the best measures of a baby's health were Kicking, Applauding, and Yawning.

Conclusion

In almost a third of cases, my colleagues are idiots and can't spell the name of the only fucking operation they have to remember the name of.

Thursday, April 17, 2008

Sometimes it's the little things that make a difference on the labor ward. The touch on your arm and a muttered "Thank you" from the mum too exhausted by her labor to speak. The Diet Coke an SHO buys you because you look so knackered. The reassuring nod from your consultant that says *You've got this*. And sometimes it's the really massive things that make a difference—like a patient's husband pulling me aside after an emergency cesarean to thank me, then mentioning that he's head of marketing for the UK operations of a large champagne house and taking my name so he can send me "a little something." I spent a week dreaming of splashing about in a gigantic champagne coupe filled to the brim with prohibitively expensive fizz, like an ostentatious burlesque act.

Today a package arrived for me at work—and I don't mean to be ungrateful, but seriously? A branded baseball cap and key ring?

Monday, April 21, 2008

Performing an elective cesarean section, assisted by a hungover medical student. With the possible exception of diathermy,* which smells deliciously like frying bacon, the sights and smells of labor-ward theaters aren't great for the morning after. Take a look at the ingredients: There's over half a liter of blood spilled, plus a tidal wave of amniotic fluid when you cut through the uterus; the baby's covered in more gunk than you'd find in the plughole of a cattery, and the placenta always smells like stale semen—none of which you really want to be faced with when your burps still taste of Jägerbomb and you're sweating rogan josh through your eyeballs. Baby delivered, and just as I was sewing up the uterus, the student fainted, face-planting right into the open abdomen. "We should probably give the patient some antibiotics," the anesthesiologist suggested.

Tuesday, May 13, 2008

At a pub quiz with Ron and a few others and one of the questions is "How many bones are there in the human body?" I'm off by about sixty, to the general

---

* *Diathermy* is essentially a soldering iron—it heats up the area you touch it on and stops small blood vessels from bleeding by sealing them off. It is important not to clean the skin with alcohol-based antiseptic before the operation, otherwise diathermy sparks can set the patient on fire.

outrage of my teammates. I try to explain myself—it's not something you'd ever be taught; there's no clinical situation where you'd actually need to know this; it's an irrelevance; I wouldn't expect Ron to be able to say how many types of taxes there are—but it's too late. I can see from the horrified looks on my friends' faces that they're trying to think back to all the times they've asked for medical advice from a doctor who doesn't even know how many bones the human body has. Three other teams got the correct answer.[*]

Monday, June 2, 2008

Prenatal-care clinic. Called in by a midwife to evaluate her patient, a low-risk primip[†] at thirty-two weeks here for a routine checkup. The midwife was unable to pick up baby's heart with the Sonicaid[‡] and so wants me to pop in. This happens fairly often, and 99 percent of the time all is well. I tend to grab a portable ultrasound machine, wheel it in like a dessert cart, quickly show the parents their baby's heart on a monitor, then wheel it all back out again, grinning like a game-show host. When they've had the agony of listening in vain

---

[*] It's 206.

[†] Primip (short for *primiparous*), meaning first pregnancy. Multip (*multiparous*) for subsequent pregnancies.

[‡] *Sonicaid* is the handheld device that you listen to babies' hearts with.

for baby's heart swoosh-swooshing, all they want is some unequivocal evidence on a screen.

This is clearly the 1 percent, though, and I can tell as soon as I enter the room. This midwife really knows what she's doing, and she looks ashen. The patient is a GP, married to an ophthalmology registrar, so we're in the rare situation where everyone in the room already knows there's something seriously wrong. I can't even manage to get out my "I'm sure everything's fine" speech before I put the ultrasound probe on.

To make matters worse, I have to call a consultant in to confirm fetal death for the notes, even though both parents know I've been looking at the four un-moving chambers of their baby's heart on the screen. She's being rational, practical, collected—suddenly in work mode, her emotional shields up as high as mine. He's in bits. "You shouldn't have to bury your child."

Thursday, June 5, 2008

The schedule has been flinging me around the hospital seemingly at random—from prenatal clinic to gynae OR to infertility clinic to labor ward to colposcopy to scanning—so everyone feels like a stranger at the moment. I've all but given up hope of seeing someone I recognize unless it's the barista handing me a latte in Starbucks.

It's especially rare to see the same patient more than

once, but on my afternoon rounds of the labor ward I see the GP I'd diagnosed with an intrauterine death in clinic earlier this week. She's now in labor, having been induced.* She and her husband seem oddly pleased to see me—a familiar face, someone who doesn't need an explanation and is already tuned in to what's happening, who can be of some comfort on such an awful, scary day.

What the hell can you say? It feels like a woeful gap in our training that no one's ever told us about talking to grieving couples. Will I make it better or worse if I talk positively about "next time"? I want to give them hope but feel like I shouldn't say it. It's an extreme version of "There are plenty more fish in the sea" after a breakup, as if babies are totally interchangeable just so long as you have one. Do I say how sad I feel for them? Is that making it all about me, giving them yet another person's feelings to consider? They'll have plenty of their own family members throwing themselves at their feet in misery; they certainly don't need this from me. How about a hug? Too much? Not enough?

Stick to what you know. I just talk practically about what will happen over the next few hours. They have a thousand questions, which I answer as best I can. This is clearly their way of coping for now, medicalizing it.

I pop back every hour or so to see how they're do-

---

* It's a terrible cruelty that if a baby dies in utero, the safest place to deliver is on the labor ward, surrounded by dozens of mothers and babies.

ing. It goes past eight p.m., and I decide to stay on labor ward until she's delivered. H is expecting me back home any minute but I lie in a text that there's been an emergency and I need to stay. I don't know why I can't just tell the truth. I lie to the patient too when she asks why I'm still here after eleven p.m. "I'm covering for someone," I say. It does feel like my presence, if not my conversational skills, are helping them a bit.

Delivery happens shortly after midnight, and I take blood samples from mum and talk through all the possible tests we can do to find a cause for the stillbirth. They opt for everything, which is understandable, but this means I have to take skin and muscle samples from the baby, the worst thing for me in this whole job. It used to upset me so much when I first started that I'd practically have to look away while I did the necessary. Now, slightly more desensitized to a thing you can never quite believe you'll ever become desensitized to, I can look. I just find it heartbreakingly sad, cutting into a dead baby. We expect them to look beautiful, perfect, unspoiled; often they don't. He's been dead a couple of weeks, looking at him—he's macerated, skin peeling, head softened, almost burned-looking. "I'm sorry," I say to him as I take the samples I need. "There we go, all done now."

I dress him again, look up to a God I don't believe in, and say, "Look after him."

Tuesday, June 10, 2008

Stopped by the police in west London. "Did you know you just ran a red light there, sir?" I honestly didn't. I'd been driving home on autopilot, utterly exhausted after a relentless night shift that included five cesarean sections. Hopefully I was paying more attention in the OR than on the road.

I explain to my frontline brothers that I've just come off the labor ward after thirteen hours. They give not a single shit, a sixty-pound fine, and three penalty points.

Wednesday, June 18, 2008

I'm no stranger to speaking in code in front of patients. Just a stray word here or there can be the difference between a patient drawing up ambitious plans to build a shrine in your honor or hysterically accusing you of plotting her demise. So we've got our equivalent of spelling out w-a-l-k-i-e-s in front of the dog or t-r-i-a-l s-e-p-a-r-a-t-i-o-n to outfox an eavesdropping five-year-old.* But it's not just patients who

---

* There are three grades of code. First, there's the formal Latin and Greek terms for conditions So, we say *dyspnea* rather than *shortness of breath* and *epididymo-orchitis* rather than *manky cock and balls*. Second, there's using a layer of euphemism. Instead of suggesting syphilis, we ask to "check the VDRL," which is the lab test involved; rather than saying HIV, we can talk about "CD4 deficiency," referring to the underlying im-

need to be kept in the dark from time to time. On this job I've also had to develop a code so Miss Bagshot can't understand me just to survive her interminable consultant ward rounds. When I need a caffeine hit I tell the house officer to "go see Mrs. Buckstar," and he pops down to Starbucks for me. Three months in and she hasn't broken this seemingly uncrackable cipher. Either that or she's turned on by my coffee breath.

Friday, June 20, 2008

I'm teaching the SHO a method of skin closure using staples that I think gives as good a cosmetic result as

---

mune problem. Third, and much more fun, are the completely made-up ones that have entered medical vocab in the last couple of decades. They generally sound credible and scientific and allow you to be frank in front of the patient without them realizing.

A few of my favorites are:

Chronic glucose poisoning—Obesity.

Incarceritis—Onset of symptoms immediately following arrest.

Q sign—Tongue hanging out of side of mouth, in the shape of a Q. Prognostically speaking, a very bad sign, though not as bad as the Dotted Q sign, where there's a fly on the tongue.

Status dramaticus—Medically well but overemotional.

Therapeutic phlebotomy—Gets better after a blood test.

Transferred to the fifteenth floor—Dead. (NB: The number should be one higher than number of floors in the hospital.)

sutures in a quarter of the time.* He does an excellent job using this technique, but I count at the end that he has used ten staples. I explain it's bad luck to close with an even number of staples and ask him to put in an extra one in the middle of the incision. I'm not superstitious—I'll happily limbo under ladders or live in a flat full of open umbrellas—but it's something I was taught years ago and have passed on to juniors ever since. Science may trump the supernatural, but once someone tells you an operative technique is bad luck, it's probably better to be safe than sorry. No one wants to be bleeped in the middle of the night because a plateful of intestines has made a surprise appearance out the front of a patient's abdomen.

Fully briefed on how to fend off this imminent crisis from the spirit world, my SHO takes the staple gun to insert the final talisman—and accidentally drives a staple deep into the pulp of my finger.

Thursday, July 3, 2008

Patient TH has been telling me for two days now that her breast pump is bugged. I've had to promise her that we'll have it investigated because when I tried to reassure her initially, she started screaming that I was in with the Russians as well. I made my fairly uncon-

---

* Materials and technique in skin closure vary surgeon by surgeon. The staplers, and indeed staples, used are a barely modified version of the kind you'd buy at Office Depot.

troversial diagnosis of puerperal psychosis[*] but failed to persuade the psychiatrists that she was sufficiently unhinged to justify an evaluation. They weren't convinced she was at risk of endangering herself or her baby. It felt rather like an orthopedic team refusing to see a patient who had a broken leg because he wasn't due to participate in the New York Marathon.

Phone call from the ER today—patient TH is currently being reviewed by psychiatry, having been brought in by the police. The Starbucks downstairs had phoned 999 after she showed up, stripped off all her clothes, stood on a table, and started singing "Holding Out for a Hero." Useful to know where the psychiatrists set the bar.

Friday, July 4, 2008

Patient NS presents to urogynae clinic for replacement of a lost ring pessary.[†] She asks if there are options

---

[*]   *Puerperal psychosis* is the nuclear version of postpartum depression—severe psychiatric symptoms in the days after giving birth; it occurs in roughly one in a thousand women.

[†]   A *ring pessary* is a doughnut of stiff plastic that goes up the vagina and keeps the internal organs, well, internal. Pessaries have existed as long as pelvic-organ prolapse, which is to say a couple of years after the first woman gave birth. Historically, a popular type of pessary was the potato—shove it up there and everything stays put nicely. Horrifyingly, the warm and moist environment is an ideal sprouting environment for root vegetables, so they would have to trim the green shoots as soon as they started bristling against their underwear.

other than the ring type, because they have a bit of "baggage" for her now. She's fifty-eight years old, and a few weeks ago was dancing at her niece's wedding, wearing "less than substantial" underwear beneath her dress. Her vigorous Macarena-ing caused the pessary to dislodge and plunge straight down onto the dance floor, then happily roll across it, eventually coming to a halt at the feet of the best man.

"What's this?" he bellowed, holding it aloft. "Has someone's pram lost a wheel? Oh! Is it some kid's teething ring?" The patient departed the dance floor and the wedding before she found out whether or not it got thrust into some poor toddler's mouth. I offer her a shelf pessary* and a sympathetic smile.

Monday, July 7, 2008

Crash call to a labor-ward room. The husband was dicking around on a birthing ball and fell off, cracking his skull on the ground.

---

* A *shelf pessary* looks like one of those hooks you put on the back of your bedroom door to hang your dressing gown on. You get it in or out by holding the hook bit, and the plate section keeps your uterus out of the public eye.

Tuesday, July 8, 2008

The phrase *roller coaster of emotions* gets a lot of airtime in obs and gynae but I've never seen the Big Dipper hurtle round its loop quite as fast as today. I'm called to the early pregnancy unit by one of the SHOs to confirm a miscarriage at eight weeks—he's new to scanning and wants a second pair of eyes. I remember that feeling only too well and scamper over. He's managed the couple's expectations very well and clearly made them aware it doesn't look good—they're sad and silent as I walk in.

What he hasn't done very well is the ultrasound. He might as well have been scanning the back of his hand or a packet of Lay's potato chips. Not only is the baby fine, but so is the other baby that he hadn't spotted. Not sure I've ever had to break *good* news before.*

---

* Twins occur in 1 in 80 spontaneous pregnancies—they're more common in IVF because you generally implant a couple of embryos a pop. Chances of triplets are 1 in 80 squared (1 in 6,400), quads are 1 in 80 cubed (1 in 512,000) and so on. Almost every complication of pregnancy is more likely the more babies you're carrying—anything of a higher order than twins is generally a bit of an obstetric catastrophe. Although I once had a patient with quads, and I seem to remember she ended up getting free nappies, clothes, baby food, and a minivan by way of sponsorship.

Thursday, July 10, 2008

Next week me and H head off for a fortnight in Mauritius to celebrate five years together. I'm excited about a bleep-free existence and hopeful I haven't forgotten how to have a relationship that isn't conducted over hurried breakfasts and apologetic texts.

The problem with being in a bubble is that it only takes one prick to burst it. It comes in the form of an e-mail from medical staffing letting me know I now need to work the middle weekend. None of my colleagues can swap with me and I don't know how to deliver babies over Skype, so I go back to medical staffing to explain my predicament. I have the kind of sinking feeling you'd have going to the headmaster's office to deny you stole licorice from the campus store with your teeth stained carbon-black.

I know colleagues who've had to cut honeymoons short and miss family funerals, so the odds were never great for them bending my schedule for a holiday. They refuse to organize a locum—their best suggestion is that I pop back to England for a bit. I don't think I'll get away with breaking this one to H by text message.

6

Registrar—Post Two

In the UK we see the skyscraper-high bills in America as the Ghost of Christmas Future unless we fight to stop the NHS getting privatized. Politicians may act dumb, but they're not, and we'll be lured very stealthily into this particular gingerbread house. We'll be promised it's only little corners of the NHS that are changing, but there'll be no trail of bread crumbs to help us find our way back through the forest. One day you'll blink and the NHS will have completely evaporated—and if that blink turns out to be a stroke, you're totally screwed.

That said, around 10 percent of the UK population have private health insurance, and they generally call on it only in nonemergency situations to get their operations a bit quicker, and the two systems exist together in relative harmony.

My opinion of private health care in the UK changed a bit during my time as a registrar. I used to be on board with it, seeing it as much like private schooling: a bunch of rich people who save the taxpayers a few quid by going off and doing their own thing, no harm done. I could always see myself doing the odd bit of private work as a consultant, one evening a week in clinic, maybe, the occasional hysteroscopy if I thought I deserved a Mercedes, perhaps a cesarean a month if I thought my Mercedes deserved a chauffeur. I knew consultants who had this life, and it didn't hurt my motivation to imagine it for myself.

And then in my second year as a registrar I started doing regular moonlighting work. I'd rather over-stretched myself on the mortgage and it felt like a sensible way of making my income do at least a rea-sonable impression of my outgoings. As free time was in short supply (and what I had of it didn't just feel like *mine* to give away), I generally took night shifts sand-wiched between normal days at work, and in order to guarantee an hour or two of sleep, I would do them in private hospitals or private wings of NHS hospitals, where the workload is a lot lighter.

These days I get asked fairly often by friends who've made much better life choices than me about whether they should have their baby privately. These are people who order from the bottom of the wine list to get a better wine or order from the bottom of the holiday-home-in-the-countryside list to get a better holiday home in the countryside, people who know that, while money might not buy you happiness, it certainly buys you nicer stuff.

This theory, it turns out, doesn't really work with childbirth. It's a shame, because if you choose to go private, you'll be dropping around fifteen grand on it, and it won't be covered by your health insurance. You'll definitely get a nicer hospital room and nicer food.

You'll certainly get an elective cesarean if you ask for it. In fact, your consultant might actively encourage you to have one. He can bill you extra for it, on top of the fifteen grand, plus he knows he won't get unexpectedly bleeped in the middle of a dinner party to pull a baby out of you. And if you start to bleed a few hours later, when your consultant is back home, the resident doctor will come along. When it was me, fine—I could deal with it, it was my day job. But I could see the rest of the roster, a lot of my colleagues in moonlighter-land normally worked as SHOs, some of them extremely junior ones, and they would be woefully underequipped to deal with a situation like that.

But what if there was a major emergency, something beyond any single doctor's capabilities? One where you needed a team of obstetricians, anesthesiologists, pediatricians, maybe even surgeons from other specialties? Then all you could do was call an ambulance, have your patient taken to an NHS unit designed to cope with this scenario, and hope she lived long enough to get there. As I say, the food's always excellent. Whether it's to die for is your decision.

Personally, I didn't ever want to risk being the doctor holding the ball when it all went wrong, so I bailed on private medicine after a few months of these shifts. Which was a bit of a shame, as I'd already decided what color uniform my chauffeur would wear.

Saturday, August 9, 2008

Nonmedical friends are always impressed when I perform spot diagnoses on members of the public; it's like an advanced level of I Spy: the lady on the bus with early Parkinson's, the man at the restaurant with lipodystrophy from HIV medication, the guy with the eye changes denoting high cholesterol, the characteristic flapping hands of liver disease, the fingernail changes of lung cancer.

But there's clearly a time and a place. "Trichomonas vaginalis," I say proudly, pointing out the telltale green discharge residue on the stripper's vulva. And just like that, I'm ruining the bachelor party, apparently.

Monday, August 11, 2008

Moral maze. Moonlighting on a unit with some private labor-ward rooms and called in by the midwife to see a woman who is pushing and has a worrying trace. I let the patient know I need to give her baby a hand coming out because its heart rate has dropped quite a bit. I tell her there's no time to wait for her consultant to come in, but it's literally my bread and butter, and everything will be absolutely fine. She understands.

Out of the room I call her consultant, Dr. Dolohov, a traditional courtesy with a private patient. He isn't very courteous in response. He says he's only a minute away and coming straight over; under no circumstances am I to deliver "his" patient. I go back into the room and prepare everything for his arrival—forceps, delivery pack, suture set. And then I decide this is ridiculous; the baby is clearly unwell and will deteriorate every moment I don't deliver it. What if he's only a minute away like every minicab is "only a minute away"? If the baby comes out compromised because of my inaction, that's my GMC license fucked. And, worse, it's a damaged baby. If this Dr. Dolohov wants to complain about me, the worst that can happen is I never work again in a hospital I now have no desire to work in.

I deliver the baby—he takes a moment to breathe but soon perks up, and cord gases[*] confirm I was right not to wait. I deliver the placenta, stitch up a graze, clean up the patient, and say, "Adam's a good name." She's calling it Barclay, naturally. Still no consultant. Moral maze correctly navigated.

---

[*] After the baby is born and handed over to the pediatricians, you take a sample of blood from the bit of umbilical cord attached to the placenta and check what's known as "cord gases." They get tested on a machine on the labor ward and definitively show how urgently the baby needed to have been delivered.

I've already changed into fresh scrubs by the time Dr. Dolohov finally appears. To give him credit, he's heard the cord gases from a midwife and gives me a huge apology. I'd have preferred it if he'd given me a huge sum of money, especially as he'll be charging the patient thousands of pounds for the delivery that *I* did, but there you go.

Friday, September 5, 2008

"Do you have a place?" asks Dr. Lockhart in morning prenatal-care clinic. It takes me a moment—we've been talking about holidays, how I've finally booked one and would be off to France with H.

"Yes . . . I mean, we've booked our tickets—"

"No! A place! Do you have a little place there?"

How deliciously out of touch he is with the life of a registrar. I can barely afford the mortgage on a tiny flat despite our two incomes; a bolt-hole in France seems as likely a next move as buying a racehorse or a time-share on the Death Star. However, this is clearly a normal thing for a consultant to have—an aspirational light at the end of the registrar tunnel.

He apologizes that he's going to have to leave clinic a little early today—in fact, he says, he should probably head out immediately.

There are fifty-two patients in clinic and I'm now the only doctor here. There may well be a light at the end of the tunnel, but the tunnel is eighty-five miles long, crammed full of impacted feces, and I have to eat my way out of it.

Thursday, September 11, 2008

I almost cry at the end of an unforgiving night shift when I see my pigeonhole has something other than a nit-picking memo about parking or hand gel; it's a lovely card from a patient. I remember her well. I repaired a tear she sustained a couple of weeks ago during a spontaneous vaginal delivery.

> *Dear Adam,*
>
> *Just wanted to say thank you. You did a fantastic job—my GP checked my stitches and said you could hardly tell I'd had a baby, let alone a third-degree tear! I'm extremely grateful to you. Thank you again.*

Everything about it is so thoughtful, the kind of thing that makes the whole job totally worthwhile. She even made it herself—a beautifully textured white card adorned with her baby's footprint in gold paint on the front. Then again, I guess she didn't have a choice—there can't be much call in Hallmark for "Thanks for mending my anus!" cards.

Tuesday, September 16, 2008

In labor-ward triage, a woman is furious that three or four people who arrived after her have been seen *before* her. "If I ever have to go to hospital, madam," one of the midwives calmly tells her, "I want to be seen last. Because that means everyone else there is sicker than me."

Thursday, September 18, 2008

My phone rings at eight p.m. I try to guess whether it's because I've forgotten to turn up for a night shift or because someone else has failed to turn up for one and I'm about to get pulled back to the ward on my invisible bungee rope. Happily, it's just my friend Lee, although he sounds rather worried. Lee is reliably my calmest, most unflappable friend, so this is alarming, to say the least. He works as a criminal defense lawyer, and I regularly hear him talking on the phone with policemen, judges, and so forth, cheerily asking things like "And was the whole body destroyed by the acid or just the skull?" and "Roughly what size of genocide are we talking?" He asks if I'm free to come over; his flatmate Terry has injured himself and Lee suspects he may benefit from going to the hospital but would value my advice. It's not far away and I'm not doing anything that can't wait, so I pop over.

Terry has indeed injured himself. From the most insignificant of actions can come the most serious of consequences, and we've gone full butterfly effect here. He cut his thumb opening a humble can of beans, severing a little artery that's currently irrigating the floor, and the top of his thumb is flapping open like a Muppet's mouth. There's even bone visible. I'm happy to provide my professional assessment that a visit to hospital is not just advised; it is both crucial and urgent. I suspect very few people in the world would disagree with me on this point. Unfortunately, Terry is one of them.

Lee pulls me into the kitchen for a moment. Terry will take quite some persuading to go to hospital—he drinks rather heavily and worries that any blood tests will show liver damage and lead to a cascade of investigations and misery he has no interest in. It would also explain why he was bleeding so heavily and why the expression "blood is thicker than water" didn't seem to apply to him.*

I spend a short while trying to negotiate with Terry. I suggest the doctors will be too concerned with the fact that half his thumb is hanging off to bother delving too far into anything else, but it's clearly not a fight I'm going to win. He won't even let me call an ambulance so the EMTs can come and assess him. I go back to Lee to formulate a plan B while Terry ruins a couple more tea towels.

Lee has a plan B, which is presented to me in the

---

* Among the liver's many and confusing functions, it produces a whole load of clotting factors, meaning that liver failure causes defective clotting.

form of a small crate of medical supplies. A year ago he took a holiday in Uganda, and the advice given to plucky travelers is to buy one of these kits before you leave and keep it with you while you're away. If you get hospitalized during the trip, they can use your equipment rather than theirs, and you'll protect yourself from some hospitals' slightly laissez-faire attitude to infection control.

Lee unseals the case, opens it out in front of me like a dodgy market trader, and asks me if I have what I need to sew Terry back up. He clearly splashed out on the deluxe package—there's probably enough in there to take out a lung. After a short while cooing over it like an auntie trying to find the hazelnut swirl in a box of chocolates, I select suture material, scissors, needle-holders, swabs, and cleaning solution; the only thing missing is some local anesthetic. Lee jokes that Terry can just bite down on a wooden spoon.

And so, five minutes later, I find myself operating on a remarkably up-for-it Terry at the kitchen table. I clean the wound, place some big deep stitches to try and stop the arterial bleeder, then start closing the thumb up in layers. The pain quickly gets a bit much for Terry to tolerate, and, eager to keep his screams to a minimum (if the neighbors pop in to check if everything's okay, this will all take some explaining), Lee hands him the wooden spoon. And it works remarkably well.

I soon close up the skin and am rather pleased with the cosmetic result. I'm not sure how receptive Terry is to my advice on wound care and removal of stitches, but I give it anyway while he shivers his thanks and reaches for a drink, resolving never to eat beans again. I quietly ask Lee about the medicolegal implications of the evening's events. He laughs and swiftly changes the subject, then packs me off in a cab with a nice bottle of rum. (Presumably Terry's.)

On the way home, I realize Terry should probably have a few days of antibiotics, given the slightly back-street nature of the procedure. I call Lee to make sure he sends Terry to the GP in the morning. I apologize for not writing a private prescription, but it's against GMC guidance to prescribe for friends and family. I can hear Lee's eyes rolling over the phone. "I think that's the least of your worries here."

Thursday, October 16, 2008

Handing over an extremely busy labor ward to a moonlighter. We've been working flat out all day, and it's not going to be a quiet night either. There are a couple of women likely to end up with sections, a couple more heading toward instrumental delivery, plus triage and ER calls Jenga-ing up. I apologize profusely to him—busy shifts are twice as difficult when you're a moonlighter and don't know the peculiarities of a hospital. I can sense there's all sorts of inner turmoil going on behind his eyes, but he says nothing.

I realize I may have made it sound a little too ghastly,

so I backpedal slightly. "Room five might deliver normally, actually, and I don't think there's anything too
urgent in the ER just now, so . . ." This doesn't seem
to have done the trick—he still looks terrified. He asks
me in broken English if he's expected to do cesareans.
I suspect he's asking whether the SHO he's on with can
operate, and I explain that she's very junior. But, no,
he's asking if he might have to do a cesarean tonight—
he's never done one before.

I ready myself for the explanation of what is clearly
a hilarious misunderstanding. Maybe he's meant to be
working as a neurology registrar and just turned up on
the wrong ward, and our real moonlighter—the one
who can actually do what needs to be done—is just
about to stroll in, blaming some confusing signage.
Nope, this guy accepted a shift from the agency as an
obstetric registrar and no one there or at the hospital
bothered to ask whether he'd ever worked in obstetrics
or on a labor ward before.

I send him home and call the consultant to ask what
to do, knowing full well the answer involves me working another twelve hours for free.

Monday, October 20, 2008

Patient HT has absolutely nothing wrong with her—
physically, at least. She's had normal blood tests,
normal swabs, a normal hysteroscopy, and a normal
laparoscopy. There's no gynecological (or any other

kind of -logical) cause for the pelvic pain she describes, and she's had no benefit whatsoever from the myriad treatments we've tried.

She still insists it's gynae. "I know my own body!" She even knows the exact treatment she would like— for us to remove all of her pelvic organs. I and various colleagues and bosses have explained at length that we don't think it will help her symptoms in the slightest, plus it would be a big operation that carries nontrivial risks, including the chance it would cause adhesions* and result in worsened pelvic pain. She's adamant it's the only answer, "as I've been saying all along," and won't contemplate any options other than ripping out all of her plumbing. Maybe she's run out of storage at home and just wants to clear some extra space?

It falls to me to finally discharge her from clinic and refer her to the pain-management service, who might eventually put her on antidepressants. This doesn't go down well, and I get everything from "I've paid taxes all my life!" to "Call yourself a doctor?" plus a list of all the people she's going to complain to, from the chief executive of the hospital to every local politician. I tell her I appreciate her frustrations, but I really

---

* *Adhesions* are bands of internal scar tissue caused by previous operations or, sometimes, infections. They can cause pain for the patient and also make subsequent operations much harder by gunking together all the organs. It's not always perfectly laid out in there like steaks and sausages on an OCD barbecue, you know.

think we've done all we can for now. She asks for a second opinion and I tell her she's already seen a large number of our doctors, all of whom were of the same opinion.

"I'm not leaving here until I'm booked in for this operation," she announces, hands folded in her lap, and she clearly means it. I don't have time to wait for Satan to put on gloves and a North Face jacket, so I decide to book her in for another appointment in a few weeks' time, throwing a colleague under the same bus I've just dodged the fare on. I've got no doubt she can, and will, waste this clinic's resources for another year or more.

Before I offer her this appointment, she screams, *"Why does no one take me seriously?"* then picks up a sharps bin* and throws it at my head. I yelp, duck, and constrict my anus to a one-millimeter bore. The bin hits the wall above my desk and a shower of virulent needles rains down around me. Somehow, like Road Runner escaping a Wile E. Coyote assassination attempt, I'm not hit by any of them and avoid catching twelve strains of HIV. A nurse runs in to see what the kerfuffle is and then goes to phone security. And with that, the patient is discharged from clinic. Next!

---

* Every office has separate bins for general rubbish, paper, plastics, et cetera, for everyone to ignore. In medical settings we also have the sharps bin—rigid plastic tubs where you dispose of used needles, blades, lancets, and the like.

Thursday, November 6, 2008

I have lost a pen. Or, more accurately, my pen has been stolen. Or, even more accurately, it has been stolen by one of the three people in delivery room five: patient AG, her boyfriend, or her mother. I wouldn't mind so much were it not a birthday present from H, were it not a Montblanc, and had I not just delivered AG's baby.

The labor itself was without serious incident, but they'd been aggressive throughout my time with them, and their feral snarling matched with the considerable tattoo count—baby excluded, for now—made me slightly reluctant to accuse them of larceny.

I guess I'm lucky to have made it this many years without something getting pinched. Colleagues have had scrub pockets picked, bags nicked from the nursing station, and lockers broken into, not to mention tires slashed in hospital car parks and even the odd physical assault.

I had a moan to Dr. Lockhart, whom I wouldn't trust to cut a patient's toenails but who is always good for a bit of advice and an anecdote. The advice was to forget it, don't get stabbed, and kudos to the patient for recognizing a decent pen. Then he got started on the anecdote.

Before his career in obs and gynae, Dr. Lockhart had worked as a GP in South London for a short chunk of the seventies. He'd celebrated getting a permanent job in general practice by buying himself a bright blue MGB convertible. The car was his pride and joy—he talked about it constantly to patients, friends, and colleagues; waxed and polished it every weekend; only just stopped short of having a photo of it on his desk. And then one day it was over, as happens with all one-sided love affairs; he finished his clinic and clocked that the bright blue MGB convertible was missing from the car park. He called the police, and they did all they could but ultimately failed to find the car. Lockhart's topic of conversation with patients, friends, and colleagues now switched to the wretched state of the world—how could someone steal his beautiful car?

One day he was telling his tale of woe to a patient who turned out to be a high-ranking member of what amounted to a local family of gangsters, and, thanks to that bizarre moral code criminals seem to hold dear, he was disgusted by this. What kind of lowlife would steal a doctor's car? Absolutely unacceptable. He said he was sure he'd be able to identify the felon and persuade him to return the car, though Dr. L of course said there was absolutely no need—the same way you would claim there was "absolutely no need" for someone to buy you an all-expenses-paid trip to the Seychelles. In other words, *Go on, then*.

Later that week, Lockhart arrived at work to find a bright blue MGB convertible in the car park, its keys on the dashboard. His overwhelming relief turned to more mixed emotions at the realization that the car had a completely different number plate and interior.

Saturday, November 15, 2008

An e-mail from Mme. Mathieu telling me, with great regret, she's refunding the rest of the term's fee for my Conversational French class because I've now missed so many lessons it's pointless coming back. E-mail correspondence with Mme. Mathieu is usually conducted entirely in French to fully immerse us in the language. This is the first e-mail I've had from her in English; she's clearly not confident I'd understand otherwise, which really rubs *sel* into whatever the French for "wound" is.

Monday, November 17, 2008

Superstition dictates you can't ever describe a shift as "quiet," much like you don't say "Good luck" to an actor or "Go fuck yourself" to Mike Tyson. Say the Q-word to a doctor and you're all but performing an incantation, summoning the sickest patients in the world to your hospital. I turn up for a locum night shift on a private obstetric unit and the registrar lets me know it should be "very quiet tonight." Before I can flick water at her and rattle off *"The power of Christ compels you!"* a few times, she tells me a high-ranking royal from a Gulf state has just delivered a baby on the labor ward, which goes some way to explaining the Oscars-level security everywhere and all the suede Ferraris outside.

As far as I'm concerned, roping off three tables in a pub for a twenty-first birthday is a bit swanky, but our esteemed guests have not only booked the entire maternity unit so there's not a single other patient around, but their consultant will be staying overnight as well, just in case. (It was fair to say the shift was quiet.)

Tuesday, November 18, 2008

Ron phoned me for some medical advice this evening. His dad has been losing a lot of weight and having midchest discomfort and increasing difficulty in swallowing. When he went to his local clinic about it this morning, the GP thought he was looking a little yellow around the gills and referred him to be seen by gastro within the week. What did I think was going on?

If I were being asked on an exam paper, I'd have said it was metastatic esophageal cancer with a survival rate of 0 percent. If I were being asked by a patient, I'd have said it was very worrying and we'd want to investigate extremely urgently to rule out the possibility of cancer. But if I'm asked by someone close to me? I said it sounded like his GP was doing everything right (true) and that it still could be nothing (definitely untrue—there was no plausible version of events where this was anything other than a very bad something). I desperately wanted it to be okay—for Ron and for his dad, who I've known since I was eleven—so I lied. You never lie to your patients to give them false hope, but there I was, doing exactly that, reassuring my mate that everything would be fine.

We're constantly reminded by the GMC not to be doctor to friends or family, but I've always just ignored that and provided them an on-call private service. Because my job makes me such a useless friend in so many ways, I guess I feel like I have to offer *something* to justify my name on their Christmas-card lists. And this is basically why we're taught not to.

Thursday, November 20, 2008

In no other job would you be expected to wear shoes from a communal supply on a "first come, first served" basis. It's like being at a bowling alley, but one where people constantly get splashed with amniotic fluid, blood, and placental tissue, and everyone's too lazy to clean the shoes afterward.

If you want your own personal white leather hospital clogs, they cost around eighty pounds, so it's previously only consultants who've splurged on them, gliding around the hospital looking like they've got giant Tylenol caplets on their feet. But now there's a new breed of shoes called Crocs—they come in bright colors, do the same job, and cost less than twenty quid. They have the added advantage of having holes in them, so you can padlock your pair together and no other bastard will get his hands or verrucae on them.

Today a notice has appeared in the changing rooms:

STAFF MUST UNDER NO CIRCUMSTANCES WEAR CROCS FOOTWEAR AS THE HOLES DO NOT PROVIDE ADEQUATE PROTECTION FROM FALLING SHARPS. A frustrated personal stylist has added underneath: AND THEY MAKE YOU LOOK LIKE A DOUCHE.*

Saturday, November 22, 2008

Called to the ER to see a nineteen-year-old girl with heavy vaginal bleeding—same old, same old. What I'm in fact faced with is a nineteen-year-old girl who has taken kitchen scissors and performed her own labial-reduction surgery. She valiantly managed to chop three-quarters of the way down her left labium minus before she called (a) it a day, and (b) an ambulance. It was an absolute mess down there, and bleeding heavily. I checked with my senior registrar that I wouldn't inadvertently be performing female genital mutilation and go to prison if I cut off the loose end and oversewed the bleeding edge. All fine, and I tidied it up. In honesty, she didn't do much worse of a job than a lot of labiaplasties I've seen.

I booked her into gynae outpatient clinic in a few weeks' time and we had a bit of a chat, emergency now out of the way. She told me she "didn't think it would bleed," to which I didn't have anything helpful

---

* Presumably the same wag who changed the sign that says WARNING! THIEVES ARE OPERATING IN THIS DEPARTMENT! to WARNING! SURGEONS ARE OPERATING IN THIS DEPARTMENT!

to reply, and that she "just wanted to look normal." I assured her there was absolutely nothing wrong with her labia; they really, honestly, did look normal. "Not like in porn, though," she said.

There's been a lot of media noise about the damaging effects of porn and glossy magazines on body image, but this is the first time I've seen it firsthand—it's horrifying and depressing in equal parts. How long until we're seeing girls stapling their vaginas tighter?*

Wednesday, December 10, 2008

This week the hospital is running a diary-card exercise.† I presume that in normal jobs, administrators monitor employees because staff are working *fewer* hours than they're paid for.

Consultants never previously spotted on a ward are writing discharge summaries for patients, working a few hours in labor-ward triage, seeing patients in the ER, all to maximize the chances of the juniors leaving

---

* The answer, as it turns out, was a year. A colleague saw a patient who'd superglued the introitus of her vagina because her boyfriend had been pressuring her to.

† During a diary-card exercise, doctors have to record their exact hours worked. But because hospitals can't (or don't want to) pay us for the time we actually work, they render the process completely meaningless. Either they lean on us to lie in the diary cards and just record our contracted hours or they throw dozens of consultants onto the wards to temporarily ease the burden on the juniors.

on time. This will continue until the nanosecond the diary-card exercise ends, of course, but for now I'm enjoying the rewards. It's my third consecutive shift leaving when I'm supposed to, prompting H to sit me down and ask if I've been sacked.

To ensure the illusion of accuracy, clerical staff from hospital management shadow a few doctors at random during their shifts. I was joined by one on a shift—or at least until 10:30 p.m., when she went home after unironically announcing she was exhausted.

Monday, December 29, 2008

Seeing a patient in gynae clinic whose GP recently started her on HRT patches and who now has some PV bleeding. I ask her how long she's been on the HRT and she lifts up her blouse and counts the patches. "Six . . . seven . . . eight weeks." Her GP hadn't explained that she has to take the old ones off.

Saturday, January 10, 2009

Percy and Marietta's wedding today felt like a huge triumph against the odds. Not one but two doctors able to get their big day off work. And the whole day too, not like my former colleague Amelia, who could only wangle the afternoon of her wedding day off and ended up conducting her morning clinic in full bridal hair and makeup to make the timing work.

The main miracle is they've managed to last this long together despite a system seemingly designed to ruin their relationship. Percy and Marietta got their training posts in different deaneries, meaning the closest hospitals they could possibly work at over the course of five years were a hundred and twenty miles apart. Rather than the two of them living together somewhere mutually inconvenient, Percy moved into awful hospital accommodations and popped back home to see Marietta when the schedule allowed, which it generally didn't.

In his speech, the best man, Rufus, a surgical trainee, compared their setup to having a partner who works on the International Space Station. It was a brilliant speech, made all the more poignant because Rufus had to deliver it between the starter and main course. As soon as the pan-seared chicken livers were wolfed down, he had to dash off for a night shift.

Monday, January 12, 2009

Asked to see a patient in labor-ward triage and repeat a PV, as the midwife is uncertain of her findings. Her findings were of cephalic presentation with cervix one centimeter dilated. My findings are of breech presentation, cervix six centimeters dilated. I explain to mum that baby is bottom-down and the safest thing to do is deliver by cesarean section. I don't explain to mum which part of the baby the midwife has just stuck her finger in to one-centimeter dilation.

Thursday, January 22, 2009

I accidentally dropped the on-call bleeper into the labor-ward macerator this evening, sending it off to a crunchy death. A feeling very similar to pissing your jeans—that wonderful warm sensation of enormous relief, followed almost immediately with *Fuck, what do I do now?*

Thursday, January 29, 2009

Waited until the radio station had moved on to the next song before making the uterine incision for a cesarean. As appropriate as Cutting Crew may be for a surgeon, I refuse to deliver a baby to the refrain of "I just died in your arms tonight."

Friday, January 30, 2009

Patient DT is twenty-five years old and has presented to colposcopy clinic[*] for her first pap smear. And her second pap smear; she has complete uterus didelphys—two vaginas, two cervices, two uteri. I've never seen this before. I perform both smears and spend a minute or two working out how the fuck to label the slides and forms, as the NHS cervical screening program isn't really equipped for this admittedly rare scenario.

She's not seen a gynecologist since she was a teenager so she has a bunch of questions for me. I admit I've never come across a case like hers before but answer the questions as best I can. She's mostly worried about future pregnancies.[†] I ask if she'd mind some questions in return. Potentially inappropriate, but we have a good rapport, and I'll probably never get the opportunity to chat to someone with the condition again.

Here's what I learned. She used to mention it to guys before they had sex, which tended to freak them out, so now she doesn't mention it at all. They apparently never notice, in any case, which is hardly surprising—most guys' knowledge of female genital anatomy is sketchy at best. Aside from the old "finding the cli-

---

[*] *Colposcopy* is a fancier way of doing pap smears—having a look at the neck of the womb for precancerous cells.

[†] She's likely to be able to get pregnant, but there's increased chance of late miscarriage, premature birth, growth restriction, and breech presentation, and she's much more likely to be delivered by cesarean.

toris" cliché, many don't seem to realize girls have a separate hole for peeing—they just think it's one great multi-functioning service tunnel. More than once I've catheterized a woman during labor only for her partner to ask if that isn't going to stop the baby from coming out.

The patient tells me she prefers having sex with her left vagina, as it's bigger (as I'd noted during examination—the right needed a smaller speculum), although she says it's nice to have an option for "different sizes of guys." I suggest that if she forgets which way round it is, the mnemonic "righty tighty, lefty loosey" would apply—though in truth she's probably very unlikely to forget which way round her vaginas are.

I recount my tale to H after work. "So it's like one of those metal pencil sharpeners at school with two sizes of hole?"

Tuesday, February 3, 2009

Last day at work before moving on to our next postings. It always feels odd to leave a job where you've watched lives begin and end, spent more hours than at your own house, seen the ward clerk more than your partner, and have your departure go all but unacknowledged—but I've hardened to it by now. There's such an extraordinary turnover of junior doctors that I understand why there's no great fanfare. As a particularly venomous matron once hissed at us,

"You are temporary visitors at my permanent place of work."

I've never once had a goodbye card, let alone a present. Until today, when I found a package in my pigeonhole from Dr. Lockhart. A card to say thank you and goodbye, and a brand-new Montblanc pen.

7

Registrar—Post Three

Eventually there comes a point where you have to decide what kind of doctor to be. Not the technical stuff, like whether you're into urology or neurology, but the more important matter of your bedside manner. Your stage persona evolves throughout your training but you generally settle on a way of dealing with patients a couple of years in and carry it through into your consultant career. Are you smiley, charming, and positive? Quiet, contemplative, and scientific? I presume it's the same decision police officers make when they decide if they're good cops or bad cops (or racist cops).

I went for a "straight to the point" vibe—no non-sense, no small talk, let's deal with the matter in hand, a bit of sarcasm thrown into the mix. Two reasons, really. It was already my personality, so there wasn't too much acting involved, plus it saves an awful lot of your day if you don't do the five-minute preamble about the weather, their jobs, and their journeys every fucking time. It sets you up as a bit distant but I don't think that's such a bad thing; I didn't really want patients trying to add me on Facebook or asking what color they should paint their downstairs bathroom.

The conventional teaching is that patients want doctors to ask open questions ("Tell me about your concerns"), then give them a variety of treatment options, from conservative to medical to surgical, so the patients can make their own decisions. Terms like *choice* sound good in theory—we all like to feel we are masters of our own destinies—but have you ever been in a buffet line where there are more than a couple of entrées? People dither, they change their minds, they look for affirmation from friends. *Is the haddock nice? How about the shepherd's pie? I don't really know what I fancy.* And all the while, your fries are getting cold. Sometimes it's best to cut to the chase and remove any room for doubt.

On the labor ward especially, I found that patients gained confidence from their doctors advocating a single management plan—you need the patient to be calm and trust you implicitly with her life and the life of her baby. Likewise in clinic, I saved countless patients delays to effective treatment by not proffering a specials board of options that were almost certainly of no benefit, just so I could say there'd been patient choice. Instead I've offered my expert opinion; the patient's choice is whether or not to take it. It's what I'd personally want if I saw a doctor myself, or even if I took my car to the garage.

But there's no hiding from the fact that a direct approach makes you a less "nice" doctor. Being trusted is much more important than being liked, but it's good to have the whole set, so I decided in my third post as a registrar—now working in a huge teaching hospital—to warm up my bedside manner. It wasn't totally spontaneous, I'll admit; someone had complained about me. It was about my clinical performance rather than my behavior, but it so totally floored me that I realized I needed to do everything in my power never to attract a complaint again, and if that involved hairdresser-style chitchat and an elbow-to-elbow smile, then so be it.

A letter arrived at home out of the blue from the hospital I'd worked at two years previously, letting me know a patient I had operated on was suing me for medical negligence. As it happens, I wasn't negligent—bladder injury occurs in one in every two hundred cesareans, and she was informed of this risk preoperatively on the consent form she signed. I'd like to think the risk of *me* injuring someone's bladder was considerably less than one in two hundred, as I'd done it only once and had many more than two hundred other opportunities to do so. I felt terrible at the time it happened but knew it had been managed well—I spotted what I'd done immediately, the urologists came to repair it straightaway, and although it must have been distressing for the patient, ultimately it resulted in nothing more than a slightly delayed discharge home. I also thought it was managed well with her afterward; I was apologetic, honest, and humble, which in this case didn't require any acting at all. The last thing you want to do to a patient is actually give them one of the complications you warn them about. *First, do no harm*—it's right at the top of the job description. But shit happens, and on that occasion it happened to her.

Messrs. Cunt, Cuntsome, and Cuntiest—solicitors of the ambulance-pursuing "no win, no fee" persuasion—took a different view. According to their expert opinion, which seemed to have been honed from skim-reading a book called *Law: Just Throw the Fucking Lot at Them and See Who Gets Back Up Again*, the trust was negligent, I'd carried out the operation well below the standard reasonably expected of me, I'd greatly extended the suffering of the claimant, and I'd delayed her opportunity to bond with her newborn child.

Unfortunately, I wasn't able to countersue for the hours needlessly spent going through old medical records and meeting with lawyers and defense unions, the damage the lawsuit inflicted on my relationship by eroding the precious little time we spent together, or the cost of the Red Bulls that kept me awake on night shifts after sleepless days of report-writing. Or the suffering *I* felt—the anxiety and guilt mounted onto an already stressful working life, the unfairness of being accused of being terrible at my job, the fear that maybe I *was* terrible at my job. I always tried my absolute hardest for every patient I saw, and it was like a dagger through my heart for anyone to suggest otherwise.

The patient almost certainly had no idea how sad and exhausting the process was for me—her lawyer no doubt smoothed his mustache, put on his best concerned face, and told her it was worth a roll of the dice in case it resulted in a nice payout*—and he was right, the hospital settled out of court, as they generally do. Maybe it's just part of the gradual Americanization of our health service that it necessarily becomes more litigious. Or maybe the patient was one of those joyless types who sues half the people she meets: the bus driver who doesn't say good morning, the waiter who forgets her side of fries, me again for writing about all this. Whatever was going on behind the scenes, it left me at my lowest ebb as a registrar—asking myself why I bothered in the first place if now even the patients had it in for me. I seriously considered jacking it all in, something that had never occurred to me before. But I didn't. I decided I would scrabble desperately around for a positive to take from it, which was to do my very

---

* It would never be the doctor ending up personally out of pocket in a situation like this. The hospital would foot the bill, or, for GPs, a medical defense organization. There can sometimes be a criminal case too if it's considered gross negligence, and this doesn't apply just to doctors. In 2016, an optometrist working at Boots was jailed for manslaughter for missing a symptom in a twelve-year-old child who subsequently died. A complaint to the GMC can run in tandem with any legal complaint, jeopardizing your license and ability to practice.

best to protect myself from any future letters on legal-headed notepaper.

"Good morning!" Adam 2.0 beamed in a typically over-running prenatal clinic.

"You taking the piss, mate?" said the patient's husband. And so my revamp lasted two days.

Friday, February 6, 2009

Patient HJ needs an emergency cesarean section for failure to progress in labor. This has not come as a surprise. When I met her on admission, she presented me with her nine-page birth plan, in full color and laminated. The whale song that would be playing on her laptop (I don't recall the exact age and breed of the whale, but I'm pretty sure it was documented to that level of detail), the aromatherapy oils that would be used, an introduction to the hypnotherapy techniques she would be employing, a request for the midwife to say "surges" rather than "contractions." The whole thing was doomed from the start; having a birth plan always strikes me as akin to having a "what I want the weather to be" plan or a "winning the lottery" plan. Two centuries of obstetricians have found no way of predicting the course of a labor, but a certain denomination of floaty-dressed mother seems to think she can manage it easily.

Needless to say, HJ's birth plan has gone right to hell. Hypnotherapy has given way to nitrous oxide has given way to an epidural. The midwife tells me the patient snapped at her husband to "turn that bullshit off" when he was fiddling with the volume on the whale grunts. She's been stuck at five centimeters dilation for the best part of six hours despite Syntocinon.* We've said we'd "give it a couple more hours" twice now, so I explain baby isn't going to come out vaginally and I'm not prepared to wait until it inevitably becomes distressed and there's a huge emergency. We're going to need to perform a cesarean section. As expected, this doesn't go down particularly well. "Come on!" she says. "There must be a third way!"

I'm loath to court a PALS† complaint from a patient who wants her delivery to be blog-post-perfect and has somehow been let down by nature. I've had a complaint in the past from a patient because I refused to allow her to have candles burning while she labored. *I don't think it's such an unreasonable request*, she wrote. About having naked flames right next to oxygen tanks.

This patient's got *Strongly worded e-mail* written all over her, so I cover myself by asking the consultant to pop by and have a quick chat with her. Luckily, Dr. Cadogan is on duty—he's fatherly, charming,

---

* *Syntocinon* (synthetic oxytocin) is an intravenous drug that increases contractions and speeds up a labor. You're meant to progress by a centimeter of dilation every hour or two, and if that's not happening despite Syntocinon, it's cesarean time.

† *PALS (Patient Advice and Liaison Service)* is the hospital's complaints department. They take "the customer is always right" to bizarre new heights and no matter how trivial the complaint, they would gladly have the doctor turn up at the patient's house carrying a bouquet of flowers and wearing a hair shirt.

and soothing, and he smells expensive, which has posh women flocking to the private ward he'd much rather be on. He soon has HJ consented for the operating theater. He even offers to do the section himself, to quiet mutterings of derision and amazement from the other staff. No one here can remember the last time he delivered a baby for free. Perhaps golf's been rained out?

He suggests to the patient that he perform something called a "natural cesarean"—I've never heard of such a thing. The operating-theater lights are dimmed, classical music plays, and baby is allowed to slowly emerge from the tummy while both parents watch. It's a gimmick and no doubt attracts a huge premium as part of his Platinum Package or whatever, but HJ laps it up. It's the first time she's looked remotely happy all day. With Dr. Cadogan out of the room, HJ asks the midwife what she thinks about "natural cesareans." "If that guy was operating on *me*," the midwife replies, "I'd want the lights turned up as high as they go."

Saturday, February 7, 2009

Missed the first half of *Les Mis* thanks to a tricky cesarean at twenty-nine weeks[*] and didn't have the

---

[*] Cesarean sections are much more difficult for premature babies. The lower segment of the uterus, which you normally cut through at full term, doesn't properly form until around thirty-two weeks. This means you have to go through a much thicker part of the uterus, making it a harder and bloodier procedure.

fuckingest clue what was going on in the second half. (Especially as the goodie, Jean Valjean, and the bad-die, Javert, essentially have the same name.)

Debriefing with Ron and the others in the pub af-terward; watching the first half didn't seem to have helped anyone else understand it either.

Sunday, February 8, 2009

Simon called to say he'd cut his wrists last night after a fight with his new girlfriend and ended up in hospital for a bunch of stitches. He's back home now and doing okay, with psychiatry follow-up arranged.

He asked if I was angry with him and I said of course I wasn't. I was actually extremely angry—that he'd done it, that he hadn't called me first so I could attempt to talk him down; surely he owed me that af-ter the hours of time I've given him? I felt guilty that I hadn't done enough—that I should have helped him better or seen it coming and stopped it. And then I felt guilty about being so angry with him.

We chatted for an hour or so and I reminded him he could call me any time, day or night. But we'd had this chat so often in the last three years, and it's miserable to think that we're no further forward than when he posted that first cry for help.

Actually, that's probably the wrong way of look-ing at it. You don't cure depression, the same way you don't cure asthma; you manage it. I'm the inhaler he's decided to go with and I should be pleased he's gone this long without an attack.

Tuesday, February 17, 2009

The emergency buzzer goes off and it's a slightly tricky situation to restore calm in. As well as the usual dozen people buzzing around, there's dust and rubble everywhere, and panic as a result. If this were an episode of *ER*, there'd be half an ambulance smashed into the room with us, but no. The midwife has pulled the emergency cord so hard, she's taken down most of the ceiling.

Thursday, February 19, 2009

It's a great shame our child-protection duties* don't extend to vetoing some of the terrible names parents saddle their unfortunate babies with. This morning I delivered little baby Sayton—pronounced "Satan," as in the king of the underworld. It's hard to believe he'll get through his school career unbullied, and yet we merrily wave him off on that journey. (Or maybe he's actually the devil and I should have just shoved him back in.)

---

* All doctors have a duty, enshrined in their GMC code, to protect children and young people from abuse and neglect by acting on any concerns they have.

At lunch, fierce discussion with my colleague Katie as to whether baby Sayton is better or worse than one she delivered called LeSanya, pronounced "Lasagna," as in lasagna.

She tells me she once pulled out a baby girl the parents named Clive, though I point out we've got a Princess Michael, so that's not particularly impressive. Another colleague, Oliver, says that where he was born, in Iceland, names must be picked from a specific list from which it's illegal to deviate. Doesn't sound like the worst idea.

Wednesday, March 4, 2009

It shouldn't be a notable event when I manage to leave the labor ward on time, but today I do and have a long-arranged dinner with Grandma. She leans over after starters, licks her finger, and wipes a dot of food off my cheek. As she licks her finger again, I realize slightly too late that it was a patient's vaginal blood. I decide not to mention it.

Saturday, March 7, 2009

"Dr. Adam! You delivered my baby!" squeals the woman behind the cheese counter at Sainsbury's. I have no recollection of her whatsoever, but her story seems to check out—that is, after all, my name and occupation. I ask about "the little one," as obviously I have no memory of the baby's gender. He's doing well. She asks me ridiculously specific questions relating to the vagina-side small talk I had with her a year ago: how I got on with building the shed, if Costco stayed open until eight p.m. on Thursdays like I'd hoped. I feel slightly guilty about the colossal mismatch in impressions we made on each other. But then again, I guess it was one of the most important moments of her life, and for me she might well have been delivery number six that day. It's a peek into what it must be like to be a celebrity, a fan asking you if you remember a meet-and-greet after a concert ten years ago.

"I'll put it through as Cheddar," she whispers to me as she weighs my goat cheese—it'll save me a couple of quid and will therefore be one of the biggest perks of the job I've ever had. I smile at her.

"That's not Cheddar, Rose," announces her supervisor as he stalks past, and my bonus evaporates.

Monday, March 30, 2009

I've just printed off a scan of their baby for some parents and am wiping the ultrasound jelly off mum when dad asks if I can take another picture from a different angle, saying, "I'm just not sure I can put this one up on Facebook." My eyebrows are en route to my hairline at these life-chronicling, self-obsessed, social-media-addicted attention seekers when I take a closer look at the photo. I see what he means; it very much appears that the fetus is wanking.

Friday, April 3, 2009

Having a drink with Ron—we're talking about his job and how he's decided it's "time to move on." I sometimes think about the idea of moving on myself, but it's a slightly alien concept when I have only one possible employer in the country. He offers to set me up with his recruitment consultant and tells me he's sure I've got plenty of transferable skills.

I hear this a lot from nonphysicians, but I don't really buy it. The feeling is that doctors are expert problem solvers who pull together a constellation of symptoms to deduce a unique diagnosis. The reality is we're more Dr. Nick than Dr. House. We learn to recognize a limited set of specific problems from patterns we've seen before—a doctor is like a two-year-old who can point and say "Cat" and "Duck" but who would struggle to identify a breeze block or a chaise longue. I strongly suspect I wouldn't last long as a management consultant by applying my problem-solving skills to a failing branch of Target.

"You should absolutely be on six figures by now,"

says Ron, texting me the contact details of his recruiter. I tell him I'll get in touch with her, but I'm not sure I want to. I'm not convinced she'll want *me* either when I outline my core competency: pulling babies and Kinder Eggs out of vaginas.

Monday, April 6, 2009

Another cesarean section—this time for placenta previa.* In the event, a very straightforward one, but everyone is quiet and focused in case it gets messy. Everyone, that is, except the dad, who is determined to engage me in pitiful banter.

"Whoa, I'm glad she's got skin covering that the rest of the time"; "This must put you off women, Doc"; something about the baby's penis and the umbilical cord—all the classics. I presume it's just because he's nervous, but it's extremely irritating and distracting, and none of his lines would even make it onto the speech bubble of a saucy seaside postcard. I "Mm-hm" at his zingers and all but say, *I'm really trying to concentrate*

---

* *Placenta previa* is a placenta that is attached at the lower part of the uterus. The implications of this are that the baby needs to be delivered by cesarean because the placenta's in the way for delivering vaginally. It also means that if mum goes into labor, it's a bit of an emergency, as the placenta is liable to shear off, with profound consequences for both baby and mother (seven hundred milliliters of blood goes through the placenta every minute, her entire blood volume in five minutes).

here. Let me deliver this baby. I didn't show up at the
conception and distract you from your pumping with
my amateur-hour repartee.

He continues, "Better not come out black, eh? Ever
had a baby come out a different color to the parents?"

"Does blue count?" I offer. Banter over.

Saturday, April 18, 2009

Patient JS is twenty-two years old and has presented
to the ER with acute abdominal pain. The ER SHO
tells me she's had a negative pregnancy test and has
been seen by the surgeons, who suspect it's probably a gynae issue. I evaluate her. She looks reasonably well—pulse a bit high, tummy a bit tender, but
walking and talking easily. Admitting her to the ward
would be overkill, but sending her home would probably be underkill. If this were a daytime shift during
the week I'd probably just squeeze her onto someone's
ultrasound list to check there's nothing sinister going
on. But it's a Saturday night and the NHS runs a skeleton service. Actually, that's unfair to skeletons—it's
more like when they dig up remains of Neolithic Man
and reconstruct what he might have looked like from
a piece of clavicle and a thumb joint.

I would generally err on the side of caution and
admit her until she can be scanned in the morning,
wasting a night of the patient's life rather than sacri-
ficing my career if I've called it wrong. It also wastes

the cost of a hospital bed, which is around the four-hundred-pound mark. I suspect the cost of an ultrasonography tech would be considerably lower than this, and you'd save at least one such admission a night, but who am I to tell the hospitals how to spend their money? Particularly when they've just decided to get rid of the beds from our on-call rooms. (Perhaps they'll save money on the bed linen housekeeping remembers to change every week or two? Perhaps they were worried morale was running a little too high? That doctors would be too alert, too on it, if they got some sleep?)

We're okay in obs and gynae—the nurse on the early pregnancy assessment unit took pity on the doctors, no doubt clocking the size of the bags under our eyes, and had a spare key cut so we could nap on a hospital bed in her unit. It's an act of charity so kind and so rare that it made my colleague Fleur cry and then scour the honors website trying to work out if the nurse would be eligible for a knighthood. It's hard to describe the joy of hearing you'll have a bed to lie in after a few night shifts spent trying to snatch some sleep in an office chair. It's a bed with stirrups, but beggars can't be choosers; I'd have accepted a bed with a grand piano dangling from the ceiling above it by a single pube if there was any chance of some shut-eye.

I suddenly realize it's also a bed with an ultrasound machine sat next to it. I check that JS is still good to walk, then take her off upstairs—if all looks well on a quick scan, she can head home, and I won't even bill the NHS the four hundred pounds I've saved them through my ingenuity.

In retrospect, it was a mistake not to tell the ER nurse I was borrowing the patient. I imagined being informed of some bit of protocol that meant I wouldn't be allowed to, and nobody's got time for that kind of argument. It was also a mistake not to book an orderly to take her up with me in a wheelchair. But the biggest mistake of all was definitely made by the ER doctor who told me the patient had had a negative pregnancy test—unless "negative pregnancy test" was the rather confusing term he used for "I have not performed a pregnancy test."

By the time we've gone upstairs, through a depressing lab-rat maze of corridors, and into my makeshift bedroom with en suite ultrasound machine, JS is looking a little peaky and a lot out of breath. Ultrasound of her abdomen shows a ruptured ectopic pregnancy, her belly swimming with blood. Instead of being where she should be, in close proximity to lifesaving equipment, she's kicking back with me in an empty part of the hospital, like we're two teenagers who've slunk off for a snog.

Half an hour of panicked phone calls later, we're in the OR, JS is a few bags of blood better off, a fallopian tube worse off, and will be absolutely fine. I have no idea what the moral of this story is.

Sunday, April 26, 2009

Called to see a patient in the ER. According to the notes she is aged thirty-five and employed in a massage parlor in a capacity one suspects doesn't involve a whole lot of massaging—at least not with her hands. She presents with a lost object in her vagina. A busy shift, so no time for too many questions, and it's legs up, lights on, speculum in, see it, grab it, remove it. Without doubt, this is the worst smell I've ever experienced. Truly indescribable—other than to say that I retch, and the nurse chaperone has to immediately leave the cubicle. I imagine every bunch of flowers in the hospital suddenly wilted. I hardly want to ask, but I need to know the culprit.

The short answer is it was the head of a Fireman Sam* bath sponge. But of course! The long answer is she realized a number of months ago her income was being seriously compromised because there were certain dates of the month when her clients didn't want to be "massaged," so she created an impromptu menstrual barrier device by decapitating Samuel. Christ knows how she explained the change in his appearance to her children—did any of them notice? Were they worried they'd be off to the guillotine next if they asked as to its whereabouts? While effective at soaking up menstrual blood from above and quite notice-

---

* Fireman Sam, should you care, is an animated firefighter from the fictional Welsh town of Pontypandy who has been a fixture of UK children's TV programming since the 1980s.

ably effective at absorbing other fluids from below, the Sam-head barrier didn't have a string to facilitate its removal. Plus it had been schnitzeled flat by her clients' pummelings over the past three months.

Actually, it's unfair to say the smell was indescribable; it's describable as three months of menstrual blood mixed with vaginal secretions and the fetid semen of assorted men, the number of whom must have run into three figures. While prescribing her some antibiotics, I let her know that no further novelty sponges needed to be executed in her honor—she could stop her periods by the more traditional method of taking the oral contraceptive pill back-to-back. I leave it to the ER to decide how to label the item within the microbiology sample bag.

Monday, May 4, 2009

Another day, another emergency buzzer or twelve. I go to perform a vacuum extraction for a non-reassuring trace, but as I'm about to Dyson the little bastard out of there, the trace improves, so I take my gloves off and hand things back over to the midwife for a normal delivery. I loiter at the back of the room to keep an eye on the trace in case it misbehaves again, but all is well and soon baby's head is crowning.

Dad is down the business end, witnessing the miracle of childbirth for the first time—awwing, cooing, and excitedly telling his wife how brilliantly she's doing. The midwife tells mum to stop pushing and start panting so she can guide baby's head out slowly and, hopefully, avoid too much of a tear. As the head advances, dad screams, *"Oh my God—where's its face?"* Mum understandably also screams, her baby's head shoots out uncontrolled, and her perineum explodes. I explain to them that babies are generally born facing downward,[*] and their baby's face looks perfect (if slightly more blood-spattered than it might have been). I put some gloves on and open a suture set.

Tuesday, May 5, 2009

Patient in prenatal clinic requests a cesarean section without a clinical indication. I explain our unit doesn't perform cesareans on request; there needs to be a medical reason because it's an operation, with attendant risks of bleeding, infection, reactions to anesthesia, and so on. Her argument was she didn't want to go through a long labor and then end up with an emergency cesarean. She obviously had me bang to rights—a planned section is much safer than an emergency one, and generally safer than an instrumental delivery too—but I couldn't say so.

---

[*] Only 5 percent of babies are born looking upward, the medical term for which is *occipitoposterior*. The cutesy-wutesy term is *stargazing*, the old-fashioned term is *face to pubis*, and the term I thought I heard as a junior SHO and then mortifyingly used for a year, until I was corrected by a colleague, is *face to pubes*.

She wasn't done trying. "Aabaat fimetoo poshtapush?" she said in her finest estuary drawl, which I eventually decoded as "How about if I'm too posh to push?" I felt mean saying no, especially as a third of female obstetricians elect for cesareans themselves—it's clearly not fair.

I was on the other side of the fence yesterday. H and I were looking to upsize mildly and were going round a flat we liked with a real estate agent. The barely twenty-year-old weasel was doing the hard sell; it's a great location, we were told—he bought his own place on the road behind. This made it all the more depressing; an embryo in shiny nylon could spare the cash to buy a flat somewhere we could barely afford. Was I in the wrong job? Or was a real estate agency like a thrift shop, where the staff got first dibs on everything that comes in?

He told us the sellers of this place had previously rejected a below-asking-price offer, but he couldn't tell me how far below asking price—it's against real estate agents' weasel-law, a code of honor among the dishonorable. I asked him if his colleagues had tipped him off about how far below asking price any other offers were when he was buying his own flat. He went a delightful shade of sun-dried tomato. "Ask me my favorite number of pounds!" he said. Turns out his favorite number was 11,500.

"Ask me why some women have cesareans," I said to the patient. I waited for her intellectual satellite delay to catch up, and she asked. I answered that some women were worried about the significantly worse long-term effects of normal deliveries on bladder and bowel continence, as it would markedly affect their lifestyle. Turns out she was too, and she is now booked for an elective cesarean at thirty-nine weeks.

Thursday, June 25, 2009

Called down to the ER around eleven p.m. to assess a patient and thumbing through Twitter while I work up the strength to see her. There's a big news story breaking, but so far only gossip-merchants TMZ have reported it. "Oh, Christ," I gasp. "Michael Jackson's dead!" One of the nurses sighs and stands up. "Which cubicle?"

Saturday, July 18, 2009

If they're updating the Hippocratic oath any time soon, they should add in a line about never mentioning you're a doctor at parties. Particularly for obs and gynae staff, where it opens up an entire hell-mouth of discussion with every woman on the planet, questions about contraception or fertility or pregnancy. I've become extremely good at being vague about what I do when I meet new people or magically changing the subject.

At a house party tonight, conversation turns to the

burka, and someone chimes in that underneath their burkas, a lot of women wear very high-end fashion, often thousands of pounds worth of clothing hidden from view. "It's true," I say. "And underneath *that* I've seen many orthodox Muslim women with Victoria's Secret lingerie and half a dozen with really elaborate pubic topiary. Initials shaved in, spirals, the lot!" Absolute silence. Then I realize that I've overdone it on the mystery. "I'm a doctor, by the way."

Tuesday, July 28, 2009

Booking a woman for an elective cesarean, and her husband asks me if there's any chance they could choose a particular date. They're a British-Chinese couple, and I know that according to the Chinese zodiac, certain days of the year are lucky or unlucky, and it's of course preferable to deliver on an "auspicious date," as it's known.

Obviously we'll try our best to accommodate this, if safe and practicable. They ask me to check for the first or second of September. "Auspicious dates?" I ask, smiling and mentally clearing a space on my lapel for an Excellence in Cultural Sensitivity badge.

"No," the husband replies. "September babies go into a different school year and perform better in exams."

Monday, August 10, 2009

"Yes, madam, you *will* shit during labor. Yes, it's completely normal. It's a pressure thing. No, there's nothing I can do to stop it. Although if you'd asked me yesterday, I'd have suggested that the massive curry you ate to 'induce labor'* probably wasn't going to help matters."

Monday, August 17, 2009

Teaching the medical students a bit of pelvic anatomy when someone from med-school administration appears with news of Justin, the missing member of the group. He won't be joining us for the rest of the term, and it sounds very much like he won't be joining the medical profession at all. Last night, he got into a fistfight with his boyfriend at a nightclub and the police were called. The police noted that Justin had a quantity of white powder on him; they suspected it wasn't Splenda and arrested him on the spot. Justin's defense was that he should immediately be released on the grounds that he was a medical student and his country needed him. This backfired ever so slightly and the

---

* Curry can't induce labor. Nor can pineapple. Nor can sex. There is no scientific evidence whatsoever for these three perennial old wives' tales. I presume they were dreamed up by the inventor of the pineapple madras when he was horny.

police contacted the medical school, accounting for his absence this morning.

The administrator leaves and no one's particularly interested in learning pelvic anatomy anymore (if anyone ever was). We have a discussion about fitness to practice among medical students and getting thrown out of the profession before you even get thrown on. Every single student asks at least one gossamer-thinly-veiled "What if a student did *this*?" hypothetical question before his or her face drains of color on hearing my answer. I regale them with the story of some contemporaries of mine who got expelled. A bunch of third-years were on a rugby tour in France, a tour that consisted of the odd game of rugby and countless hours of drinking games. The most inventive of these games involved visiting local hostelries and making Very Bloody Marys. They would order large measures of vodka from the bar, return to their tables, produce needles and syringes, venesect each other, squirt blood into each other's vodkas, and then chug them down. The gendarmerie point-blank ignored the rule of "what goes on tour stays on tour" and responded quite urgently to the bar staff's concerns about all the discarded needles on their premises, arresting the students and informing the university. My tutorial group seemed happy that this was an expulsion-level offense, although one raised the mitigating factor that it was pretty impressive for a group of third-years to be able to draw blood.

"Poor Justin" still seemed to be the prevailing feeling amongst them. My suggested "Poor Justin's beaten-up boyfriend" fell on fairly deaf ears.

"I just can't believe it," one girl says with a loud sigh. "Justin's *gay*?"

Wednesday, August 19, 2009

Moral maze. Working my way through the day's elective cesareans. This one is for breech presentation—I cut through the uterus and the baby quite clearly isn't breech. Fuck. I should have scanned the baby before I started—you're always meant to, just in case the baby has turned since the last ultrasound. Which it never has. Except today.

My choices are as follows:

(a) Deliver the magical revolving baby and confess to the patient I've done a completely unnecessary cesarean section, scarred her abdomen, and confined her to hospital for a few days when she could have had a normal delivery.
(b) Deliver the baby and pretend it was breech— this would involve lying in the notes and persuading my assistant and scrub nurse to perjure themselves by colluding.
(c) Stick my hand inside the uterus, rotate the baby, grab a leg, and deliver it breech.

I choose (a) and fess up to the remarkably under-standing patient, who I suspect actually wanted a cesarean. Then it's time to fill in the clinical-incident form and tell Dr. Cadogan. He's very nice about it and says at least I'll never forget to scan a patient before a section again.

He also makes me feel much better by telling me about an unnecessary section he'd once done as a ju-nior trainee. Baby wasn't coming out with forceps, so he performed an emergency cesarean. Unfortunately, when he got inside the abdomen, the baby had some-how delivered vaginally in the meantime.

"How did you explain *that* to the patient?" I ask.

There's a pause. "Well, we weren't always quite so honest with the patients back then."

Thursday, August 20, 2009

I obtain consent from patient YS for a termination of pregnancy—an unplanned, unwanted pregnancy in a twenty-year-old student following condom failure. We discuss alternative methods of contraception and cor-rect condom usage.* I identify an error in her technique.

---

* I performed a large number of TOPs in this job, as a lot of the other junior doctors had objections for ethical or religious rea-sons (or pretended to, because they were work-shy bastards). No one's first choice of a way to spend a morning, but a necessary evil, and as a result I developed excellent surgical technique for ERPC—the near-identical surgical procedure required follow-ing certain miscarriages. By now I could probably vacuum the

I'm as big a fan of recycling as the next man, but if you turn a used condom inside out and put it back on for round two, it's probably not going to be that effective.[*]

Tuesday, October 20, 2009

We're one registrar down in prenatal clinic, so I'm sailing this shit show alone. I saw thirty patients in morning clinic, which finished at three p.m., two hours after my afternoon clinic was meant to have started.

All the patients I see are pissed off, and rightly so—they've been sitting in a waiting room for four hours, crotchety as a pen of wet hens. Safe to say my sincere apologies and not-my-faults don't count for much while they grunt their way through their appointments. I strongly suspect if I were a pilot and my

---

stairs through my letter box if needed. This patient didn't want to raise a child, and we live in a civilized society. According to the letter of the law (the 1967 Abortion Act, to be precise), in the UK two doctors need to agree that continuing with a pregnancy would be damaging to the patient's mental health, but in reality that covers any unwanted pregnancy. In this case the patient had attempted to take reasonable precautions against getting pregnant. Used correctly, condoms can be 98 percent effective, but frequent mistakes include late application, early removal, and incorrect lubrication, so it's always good to check they're being used properly.

[*] A couple of years later, I encountered an example of condom failure where the guy thought that because a condom was coated inside with spermicide, and he didn't really like the feeling of them, he could roll it on to coat his cock with spermicide, then take it off before sex.

copilot didn't turn up, the airline might find a better solution than "Plow ahead and see what happens."

Seven p.m. and two patients from the finish line, I have to make an urgent psychiatric referral for someone who's had a relapse of severe anorexia nervosa at thirty weeks. And she's eaten more than I have today.

Wednesday, October 28, 2009

I need to admit a woman for pelvic inflammatory disease so she can receive intravenous antibiotics. Unfortunately, she doesn't want to receive any because she thinks I'm in the pocket of the pharmaceutical industry, so we've reached a bit of a stalemate. We talk through her concerns. It turns out this is a very recent worry, as she read something about it on Facebook yesterday.

Yet another mark against technology, as far as I'm concerned: the trust have finally acknowledged we're in the twenty-first century and digitized our radiology system, doing away with all light boxes and physical printed X-rays. Instead, we can now access them from any computer in the hospital. Unfortunately, the system has been broken since they installed it, thereby putting our practice back in the nineteenth century, before the introduction of X-rays.

Patients frequently attend clinic with reams of articles they've googled, printed out, and highlighted, and it's pretty tedious spending an extra ten minutes per patient explaining why a blogger in Copenhagen who uses a pink-hearts WordPress theme might not be a reliable source of information. Of course, if it weren't for Google, I wouldn't be able to send a patient off for a urine sample and then look things up in a panic.

Today, technology is serving up conspiracy theories. The patient asks me to prove I'm not being bribed by drug companies. I point out that the particular antibiotics I want to put her on cost a matter of pennies and that drug companies would probably be furious with me for not choosing something more expensive. She doesn't waver. I point out that the antibiotics I've prescribed are generic, that I'm not pushing a specific company's product. She's still unmoved. I point out that I drive a five-year-old Peugeot 206, so I'm probably as far out of anyone's pocket as possible. "Fine," she says and agrees to the antibiotics.

Wednesday, November 4, 2009

Patient TH is an accountant in her midthirties who has been diagnosed with an ectopic pregnancy. She is a candidate for medical management using methotrexate,[*] and she's keen to do so and avoid surgery. I consent her

---

[*] Certain patients with ectopic pregnancies can be managed with methotrexate if they're medically well and the ectopic is small. It's a pretty nuclear drug that attacks rapidly dividing cells, meaning it's effective at dissolving the ectopic pregnancy and can also be used in chemotherapy.

for receiving the drug and talk through the follow-up procedure. I explain the possible side effects and the various dos and don'ts while she's on treatment, emphasizing that she must use effective contraception for the next three months and abstain from sex altogether for the first month after treatment. She pauses to consider this before asking, "How about anal?"*

Wednesday, November 18, 2009

Visiting Ron's dad in hospital. He looks terrible, jaundiced skin stretched tight over jutting bones. A road map of blood vessels is visible across his face where his body has burned away every single fat cell, throwing all its energy into fighting a cancer it has no chance against. "I wish people didn't have to see me like this," he says. "We'll be spending a fortune on the undertakers making me look nice afterward—can't you just wait a few more months?"

He's in hospital for an esophageal-stent insertion so he can continue to eat and drink, to make his final chapter as comfortable as possible. The retired engineer in him is fascinated by the mechanism of the stent, a self-expanding metallic mesh, strong enough to push back the tumor and open up his gullet. "Wouldn't have been possible twenty years ago," he says, and we

---

* If you're interested, the answer is "Yes, even anal." There's still a risk of the ectopic pregnancy rupturing, so we try to avoid any banging around in that neck of the woods.

talk about being lucky to live in this current blink of civilization's eye. "Do you think they'll be able to cure cancer twenty years from now?" he asks. I can't work out whether saying yes or no would be more comforting. I deflect with "I only know about vaginas, pal," and he laughs.

Next question. "Why do we always say that people lost their battle with cancer and never that cancer won its battle against them?" He keeps making jokes—to be fair, he's done it the entire time I've known him. I find it uncomfortable for the first few minutes of my visit, but I'm soon genuinely enjoying a morning I'd been dreading. It's a kind and clever move—it doesn't just make it easier for his friends and family when they visit, it also means we'll remember him as he always was, diminished physically, maybe, but not in personality.

Thursday, December 10, 2009

A poignant vacuum-extraction delivery—it's a mum I saw in infertility clinic at the start of this job. I feel like holding the baby aloft like it's Simba and blasting out my best "Circle of Life." While I'm patching her up, I ask her about the fertility treatment—turns out she got pregnant without any treatment the week after our appointment. Still, I'm taking it.

Thursday, December 17, 2009

Tragically, domestic abuse in pregnancy is still respon-sible for the deaths of mothers and babies every year. Every obstetrician has a duty to look out for it. This is often difficult, as controlling husbands are likely to attend clinics with their wives, denying them an op-portunity to speak up. Our hospital has a system to help women disclose abuse—in the ladies' room, there is a sign that says IF YOU WANT TO DISCUSS ANY CON-CERNS ABOUT VIOLENCE AT HOME, PUT A RED STICKER ON THE FRONT OF YOUR NOTES,* and there are sheets of red-dot stickers in every cubicle.

Today, for the first time in my career, a woman has dotted a few red stickers on her notes. It's a tricky situ-ation, as she's attended clinic with her husband and two-year-old child. I try and fail to get the husband to leave the room. I call in the senior midwife and consul-tant, and between us, we get her alone. As gently as we interrogate her, it doesn't do any good; she's clamming up—scared, confused. After ten minutes we establish that the red dots were the early artistic efforts of her two-year-old, who stuck them on the notes when they went to the bathroom together.

---

* In the UK, pregnant patients carry their maternity notes with them in case they have an emergency and need to go to a hospi-tal other than their usual one.

8

Registrar—Post Four

During my career as a doctor, for every "Would you mind having a look at this [lump/rash/penis]?" I heard off-duty, there was always one "I don't know how you do it." This generally came from people who wouldn't qualify for jury service, let alone for medical school, but it's still a valid point. It's a difficult job in terms of hours, energy, and emotion, and from the outside a pretty unenviable one.

By the time I was six years deep into medicine, the shine had definitely rubbed off the surface. On more than one occasion my finger had hovered over the metaphorical "Fuck it" button—days where things had gone wrong, patients had complained, schedules had changed at the last minute—and my resolve wavered. Not quite enough to start circling the jobs page of the paper, but certainly enough to wonder if I might have any long-lost millionaire aunts on their way out.

But there were two things keeping me there. First, I'd worked long and hard to get as far as I had. Second—and I realize this might sound a bit earnest—it's a privilege to be allowed to play such an important role in people's lives. You may be an hour late home, but you're an hour late home because you stopped a mother bleeding to death. You may have had forty women in a prenatal clinic designed for twenty, but that's forty women relying on you for the health of their babies. Even in the parts of the job you hate—for me it was urogynecology clinic, a bunch of grannies with pelvic floors like quicksand and their uteri stalagtiting into their thermals—each decision you make can immeasurably improve someone's quality of life. And then a patient sneezes, you have to get a mop and bucket, and you wish you'd opted for a career in accounting.

You may curse the job and the hours, own voodoo effigies of the management, and even carry a vial of ricin on you at all times in case you ever meet a health minister, but on an individual basis, you really care for all the patients.*

I must have been in this kind of upbeat mood in my fourth registrar posting when I accepted an invitation to represent medicine at my old school's careers fair. It involved a morning sitting behind a table while a bunch of gangly sixteen-year-olds lumbered around

---

* Except the ones who try to sue you.

and asked me questions about my job. Or, as it turned out, mostly asked a bunch of other people questions about their more interesting and better-paid jobs. My table definitely looked the least appealing—everyone else had stacks of leaflets and bowls of pens, sweets, and key rings. People at the Deloitte table were even handing out doughnuts, which felt a bit like cheating. What should I have brought to entice people into a career in medicine? Toy stethoscopes? Amniotic-fluid smoothies? Diaries with all your weekends, evenings, and Christmases handily crossed out?

The students who did speak to me were clever, driven, and erudite—I'm sure they would have all breezed into medical school if they chose to—and I found myself spending a lot of time discussing what's bad as well as good about the job. Even though I felt protective of my profession, particularly with the other tables around, Christ knows we need people to go into it with both eyes open. So I told them the truth: the hours are terrible, the pay is terrible, the conditions are terrible; you're underappreciated, unsupported, disrespected, and frequently physically endangered. But there's no better job in the world.

There's infertility clinic: helping women get pregnant after years of trying, women who've all but given up hope—it's difficult to explain how special that feels. It's something I'd happily do on my own time and for free (which is handy, as I frequently did—those clinics ran over by hours). And the labor ward: a true roller coaster, by which I mean everyone generally ends up alive and well despite the fact it seems to be against the very laws of nature. You dart from room to room, delivering any baby who gets sick or gets stuck, making an indelible mark on the lives of these patients. A low-grade superhero—your utility belt holds a scalpel, some tongs, and a wipe-clean Dustbuster.

The careers on the other tables had their obvious draws—the principal one being a shit-ton of cash every month—but there's no feeling like knowing you've saved a life. Not even that, half the time; just knowing you've made a difference is enough. You go home—however tired, late, and blood-spattered—with a spring in your step that's hard to describe, feeling like you have a useful part to play in the world. I said this little speech about thirty times, and by the end of the morning I felt like I'd been through rigorous couples therapy—talking all the problems out, realizing the spark was still there after all.

I felt uplifted as I left the school hall, actively looking forward to hitting the labor ward on Monday. What an honor it is to do this job—even if it is significantly worse than the sum of its parts. I stole a Deloitte doughnut and headed home.*

And the next time someone asked me, "Seriously, how do you do it?" I truly knew what the answer was. Although the reply I generally gave was "I like operat-

---

* Full disclosure: I did also take a leaflet about their graduate-entry program.

ing on strangers' vaginas," which at least ended the conversation quickly.

Friday, February 5, 2010

Doing an elective C-section for a woman who's had three previous sections—her abdomen is absolutely rock-solid with adhesions. I call my senior registrar in to help and demote the SHO to a spectator role. Scar tissue means that bowel is matted to bladder is matted to uterus is matted to muscle is matted to God knows what. It's like ten pairs of headphones have become tangled together and then the whole thing has been encased in concrete.

The senior reg tells me it will take as long as it takes—we just need to be slow and methodical. Better that it takes three hours than the patient needs her bowel repaired and spends an extra week in hospital. We assume the pace of an arthritic archaeological dig. Every time it gets a bit easier and I speed up, the SR puts his hand on mine and I slow right down again.

Eventually there's nearly enough space to make the cut and deliver the baby—just one last loop of bowel to gently encourage away from the uterus. I'm in the process of peeling it off when the unmistakable fetid stench of bowel contents fills the operating theater. Shit. Literally. And we were so close.

The SR tells me to deliver the baby—he'll pop out

and bleep a bowel surgeon over to repair the damage.* My SHO interrupts sheepishly. "Sorry, guys—that was *my* bowel."

Saturday, February 6, 2010

I meet Euan, a friend from the university dorms, and his wife, Milly, for lunch in town—they're feeding me in return for picking my brains about fertility issues. The mains arrive and I switch from reminiscence mode to doctor mode. "So. How long have you been trying, then?"

"Seven months and two weeks," replies Milly robotically, like an ATM dispensing a tenner. She's weirdly precise.

In fact, *weird* and *precise* would prove to be her watchwords, as she then dips into a tote bag to produce a folder that she passes to me, stony-faced. I am clearly being granted sight of a document of colossal importance. I flick through page after page of spreadsheets; it takes me a moment to absorb the sheer horror of her magnum opus. This is a database of every time they've had sex since coming off contraception alongside the dates of Milly's cycle and, distressingly,

---

* To test for a bowel perforation, you use a method that's remarkably similar to locating a hole in the inner tube of a bike tire: you fill the abdomen up with water and pump air through the patient's anus until you can see where the bubbles are coming from.

the length of the session and who was on top. Quite why this was documented in such detail I have no idea, unless it was a deliberate attempt to suppress my appetite and keep the lunch bill down.

I'm totally distracted for the rest of the meal, unable to shake thoughts of my ex-flatmate's sexual positions and durations and him clambering on and off, or out from under, with the regimented duty of a workhorse. I manage to collect myself long enough to offer them some half-decent advice on giving up coffee and alcohol, the blood tests they should get from their GP, the point where they need a referral to an infertility clinic.

"Is it worth keeping the diary going?" asks Milly. "Oh, definitely," I say—partly so they don't think they've needlessly shown me a sex almanac and partly to give some poor infertility registrar a good giggle in a few months' time.

Tuesday, February 9, 2010

Today, as I was making a perineum look slightly more like a perineum after a forceps extraction, the midwife asks mum if we can give her baby a vitamin K injection. The patient treats us to some tabloid-newspaper sensationalist scare-story quackery—except it appears that this woman may have been holding her paper upside down.

She declines the vitamin K because "vaccines give you arthritis." The midwife patiently explains that vitamin K isn't a vaccine, it's a vitamin that's very important to help with baby's blood clotting. And it doesn't cause arthritis—maybe she's thinking of autism, which also isn't caused by vaccines. Which this injection isn't.

"Nah," the mum says. "I'm not taking any chances with my baby's health."

Sunday, February 14, 2010

First Valentine's Day spent with H in four years. I suggest that, Valentine-wise, going out with a doctor is like having your birthday on the twenty-ninth of February.

A lovely Thai dinner at the Blue Elephant restaurant. At the end of the meal, the waiter brings over a pair of heart-shaped sweets in a beautifully carved wooden box. I eat mine whole. Turns out it was actually a candle.

Tuesday, February 16, 2010

Husband and wife are both in tears at the news that baby will need to come out via the sunroof for failure to progress in labor. The main sadness seems to be the husband's slightly odd obsession with being the first person to touch the baby. There isn't much time to muse upon why he might want to do this—perhaps he wants to break an enchanted spell or has superpowers he needs to transfer to his offspring—but he is really most insistent. Isn't there a way he can still be the person who touches her first? If he lifts her out at the end of the cesarean, maybe?

He would definitely faint, vomit, or both at what it looks like inside an abdomen: a casserole of flesh and giblets cooked up by someone irrevocably insane. Besides, it takes most trainees a good few sections before they can get a baby out by the head—unless he can quickly practice by scooping cantaloupe melons out of a swamp one-handed? Plus no one seems to realize there's a whole tricky ritual that takes time to learn, namely getting scrubbed and then into gown and gloves. Gloves! "How about if we pass baby straight to you?" I suggest. "We'll be wearing gloves, so you'll be the first person to actually touch her."

Sold.

Thursday, February 25, 2010

The emergency buzzer goes off in the labor ward. The whole team runs down the corridor and none of us can see a room with a flashing light outside.

You'd think they might come up with a more high-tech system, given that lives are at stake, but we're stuck with the airplane-passenger-call setup. One person presses a button, the entire place hears a piercing beep every couple of seconds, and then the cabin crew/

obstetric team has to traipse up and down looking for a light until they find whoever pressed it and can turn the noise off. If only I could swap medical emergencies for something as serene as refilling someone's G and T or a terrorist saying he's going to blow up the plane.

The alarm is still going and, with precious time draining away, we decide to go from room to room, checking in on every single laboring patient. Clearly one of the lights has broken.

No one seems to be having an emergency. Where else is there? Changing rooms, labor-ward ORs, restrooms, anesthesia rooms, tea room—we split up like Scooby-Doo and the gang to cover every inch of the ward. Nothing. A literal false alarm. Aside from the fact it's deafeningly loud, every single member of staff is conditioned to react to this sound by leaping into action. It's too unsettling for background noise, much like if the radio started playing an air-raid siren.

We call engineering. Some bloke comes up and fucks around uselessly with a box on the wall for ten minutes. They'll get someone over to fix it tomorrow, apparently—until then we have the choice of a constantly blaring alarm or no alarm system at all. We summon Professor Carrow, the on-call consultant, and he's furious. Mostly because he's spent the last decade successfully avoiding walking onto the labor ward during his shifts and also—as he points out to the engineer—this counts as an extremely serious clinical incident. Lives are being endangered and the company needs to come out immediately to resolve it. The

engineer mutters he'll do his best, but no promises—
and besides, what happened on labor wards a hundred
years ago, before emergency buzzers?

Professor Carrow fixes him with a zero-degree Kel-
vin glare. "One in twenty women died in childbirth."

Wednesday, March 3, 2010

I'm putting in the last of the skin staples after an uncomplicated elective cesarean when the scrub nurse
announces there's a discrepancy in the swab count—
one's unaccounted for.* Don't panic, we tell ourselves, panicking. We check on the floor and inside the
drapes—no swab. We riffle through the placenta and
blood clots in the clinical-waste bin like it's the world's
most horrific grab bag—no swab. I call in Dr. Fortescue, today's on-call consultant, to make the decision
as to whether we reopen the patient or send her for an
X-ray.†

Dr. Fortescue decides we should reopen, and we

---

* For every operation, an inventoried set of instruments are used,
and they are counted meticulously in and out. Swabs are packed
together in stacks of five, and at the end of the procedure, the
scrub nurse makes sure that the total number of discarded
swabs is a multiple of five so we know that none have been left
inside the patient. (Unless five have somehow been left inside
the patient.)

† Every swab has a radiopaque thread running through it that
shows up on X-rays as a line. A bit unimaginative—I'd have
gone for a radiopaque *Whoops!*

wait for the anesthesiologist's epidural top-up to take effect. The consultant tells me a story from a few years ago: An elderly woman presented to him in clinic complaining of lower abdominal pain. After performing various other investigations, he sent her for an X-ray. The principal finding was the presence of a spoon in her abdominal cavity. After he'd asked various pertinent questions—"Have you ever eaten a spoon?," "Do you stick spoons up your vagina or rectum?"—it seemed unlikely the origin of the object would be discovered. But it was causing her pain and needed to be removed at open surgery, under general anesthesia.

Sure enough, at surgery, nestled among her intestines and other gizzards, was a dessert spoon. On removal, its only notable features were a number of scratches on the rear surface and the words PROPERTY OF ST. THEODORE'S HOSPITAL stamped onto the handle. Dr. Fortescue saw her on the ward postoperatively and they were each equally baffled as to how the spoon had somehow managed to backpack its way from St. Theodore's into her abdominal cavity. Her last contact with the hospital, save for their spoon stirring her innards like a risotto, was a cesarean section back in the 1960s. Some correspondence with St. Theodore's followed in which they firmly denied the routine surgical implantation of spoons but were able to dig up the patient's notes. They were unrevealing, spoon-wise—it seems very few doctors who empty containers of cutlery into patients' stomachs are going to document it—but they did provide the name of the surgeon. The gentleman was long since dead, but Dr. Fortescue was eventually able to speak to someone who trained under him to ask if his old boss was in the habit of breaking mid-cesarean for a spot of baked Alaska. Amazingly, this revealed the explanation. The surgeon in question routinely used a sterilized dessert spoon when sewing up the rectus sheath* to protect underlying structures. On this occasion the spoon had clearly fallen in, and he'd just decided "Sod it" and plowed on.

Our anesthesiologist calls over that we're good to proceed, and as I start to remove the skin staples, a midwife runs into the OR telling us to stop because the swab has been found: the baby was holding it. Much relief all round, except from the scrub nurse who has been subjected to half an hour of unnecessary stress and bin-searching. "The thieving little cunt," she says—not seeing that directly behind the midwife is the swab in question, held by the baby in question, held by its father.

Thursday, March 18, 2010

The ER bleeps me urgently—a woman is delivering at twenty-five weeks. Myself, SHO, anesthesiologist, and midwife peg it down to the ER with the neonatal

---

* The *rectus sheath* is a fibrous layer underneath the abs; when you sew it back up, you need to be careful not to accidentally nick any of the underlying organs.

team following closely behind, wheeling all their para-phernalia. The woman's huffing and puffing and in a terrible state; the anesthesiologist gives her some pain relief. The midwife can't pick up a fetal heartbeat with the Sonicaid—not good.

I examine the patient. She's not actively delivering. In fact, her cervix is long, hard, and closed—she's not in labor at all. This is odd. I ask where she's followed for this pregnancy and she says it's here. Someone looks her up on the computer and there's nothing, not that this is unusual. The computer denies knowledge of almost every patient—we'd be better off with tarot cards.

One of the ER staff scrambles to find me an ultra-sound machine and I ask the patient when she had her most recent scan. Last week. This hospital, right? Yep. On the fifth floor? Yep. Ah, I see. I send the anesthe-siologist, midwife, and pediatricians away. Any scans for patients here happen on the ground floor of this *three*-story hospital.

The ultrasound machine appears, and luckily, given I've just sent away the rest of the team, there's no baby—just some distended loops of bowel making her look pregnant-ish. If you squint.

"But where's the baby? Where's it gone?" she screams to a packed and no doubt fascinated ER. I tell her my colleagues will be along shortly to explain, then ask the emergency doctors to kindly contact psy-chiatry to take over her management. I scoot over to the coffee shop for a sit-down and a quiet reflection on what I've just experienced. I'm cross that other patients have been potentially endangered by her wolf-crying dragging so many clinicians away from the labor ward. I'm baffled as to what she thought was going to happen—she knew we would figure it out, right? And I'm sad for her—what kind of traumas and demons have taken her to a place where she does this? Hopefully my friends in psychiatry are currently giving her the help she needs.

Shame on me for thinking I'd be able to get through a whole coffee undisturbed. I'm suddenly fast-bleeped to the labor ward and run there as quickly as I can.

"Room four!" shouts the senior midwife as I wheeze onto the ward. It's the woman from the ER, huffing and puffing away again. She's clearly not giving up so easily and has absconded from the ER before her psychiatric eval to try her luck elsewhere.

She sees me and looks extremely pissed off, her parade well and truly rained upon.

Saturday, March 27, 2010

A nice evening out with a few old med-school friends to persuade ourselves that our lives are fine, despite significant evidence to the contrary. It's nice to catch up, even if it needed to be rearranged seven times.

After dinner, we end up at the med-school bar, and then for some reason, perhaps muscle memory from the last time we were there, we start playing a drinking game. The only game we can all remember the rules to is "I Have Never." It descends into therapy: All six of us have cried because of work, five of us have cried while at work, all of us have been in situations where we've felt unsafe, three of us have had relationships end because of work, and all of us have missed major family events. On the plus side, three of us have had sex with nurses, one of us while at work, so it's not all bad.

Monday, April 19, 2010

Dr. Burbage, a consultant, has taken two weeks' compassionate leave because one of her dogs has died. Much ridiculing in the labor-ward coffee room. I come to her defense, to everyone's surprise, not least my own.

Dr. Burbage despises me—she decided I was hateful the moment she met me and hasn't budged from this standpoint. When I asked if I could get away from clinic early one evening for an anniversary dinner (earlier than clinic was going to end, not earlier than I was contracted to be there), she told me I should stay on the grounds that I'd "find it easier to get a new partner than a new job." On a different occasion, she told me that if I expected to work in diabetic prenatal clinic, where I'd have to speak to patients about their diet, I'd need to have some self-respect and lose some weight (my BMI is 24). She slapped my hand in the operating theater for holding a retractor incorrectly and told me off for using blasphemy after I said "Damn." She shouted in front of a patient that I was an idiot and needed to go back to med school.

And yet I'm defending her in front of my colleagues. Why make fun of someone for being upset? Surely this is cause to respect her; she knows everyone will find out her tough exterior was just that, an exterior. Shouldn't we feel sorry for someone who has so little else in her life that she can be so totally floored by the death of her pet? Grief is grief—there's no right way and no normal. Mumblings of "Maybe" all round, and I wander off, having thoroughly suffocated that conversation with the pillow of my compassion. Two weeks for a dead dog, though—the woman's fucking nuts.

Wednesday, April 21, 2010

One of the medical students saw me after a tutorial and asked me if I wouldn't mind taking a look at his penis. I did mind but didn't really have much choice—it presumably takes quite a lot of nerve to ask one of your teachers to look at your dick. (Except in porn, where it seems to happen fairly regularly.) I took him into a side room and put on some gloves for the illusion of professionalism. He told me his penis was bruised and he'd had trouble urinating since last night.

It seemed there were certain elements of the story he'd omitted; his cock looked like an eggplant that had been attacked by a tiger—swollen, purple, and with deep oozing gashes down its entire length. On further questioning, I learned he was boasting to his girlfriend last night about the strength of his erections and announced to her that its throbbing robustness could stop the rotary blades of a desk fan. His hypothesis was monumentally incorrect, and the desk fan proved the clear winner.

I suggested he present to an ER—a couple of the wounds needed closing and I suspected he might need catheterization until the swelling died down. And actually, maybe he should go to a different hospital's ER unless he fancied being known to his colleagues for the rest of his time here as Cock au Fan.

Thursday, April 22, 2010

Perform my first cervical cerclage,[*] under the supervision of Professor Carrow. In pretty much any other procedure, the consultant supervising you can slam his foot on the metaphorical dual controls at any point

---

[*] *Cervical cerclage* is the treatment for cervical incompetence—a slightly horrible, cervix-shaming term for when the neck of the womb opens far to early in the pregnancy, causing late miscarriages or very preterm births. The cerclage stitch is inserted during the first trimester of pregnancy and hopefully holds the cervix shut until just before full term.

and stop you doing too much damage. But cerclage is all on you—they can talk you through it, but the tiniest slip with your stitch, anything but the steadiest hand, and you can rupture the membranes and end the pregnancy, doing exactly what the procedure is trying to prevent. And there's no way to practice the technique at home, like the way we learned to close wounds as house officers by cutting into an orange and sewing it back up.

Patient SW lost her first pregnancy at twenty weeks and is now thirteen weeks into her second. Carrow tells me to take it nice and slow, as steadily as I can. I'm aware that any shaking of my hand is magnified tenfold at the other end of the long needle-holding forceps, up by her cervix. Deep breaths, blink the sweat out of my eyes, one stitch, two, three, four, done. Got away with it.

I think it's the first time I've changed into a fresh pair of scrubs because my own sweat was the bodily fluid soaking me. It occurs to me scrubs are probably that shade of blue so patients can't see your sweat marks—a calm and professional demeanor is all well and good until the rapid darkening of your underarms betrays you.

Later, I realize there actually would be a way to practice the exact kind of small motor skills I need ahead of next time. I text my mum to ask if she by any chance still has that game of Operation tucked away in a drawer.

She replies to say she's found it. She also has a Magic 8-Ball, she tells me, in case I need it for my diagnoses.

Saturday, April 24, 2010

Moral maze. Patient AB is in labor and has a non-reassuring trace. She's on her third midwife of the shift, having hurled racist abuse at the first two (black) midwives who had been looking after her. One more episode like that, she's been warned, and she'll be kicked off the labor ward. My SHO has reviewed the CTG and advises me that AB needs a cesarean section. Because I'm not entirely sure of the legality of following through with the threat to boot her out, the Indian SHO and I choose to ignore the fact that the patient has made racist comments to *her* too.

On assessing the patient, I agree with the SHO—C-section it is. I transfer her to the OR and decide to stay tight-lipped about the fact I'm Jewish. The operation is straightforward, and a little boy is delivered safely (presumably to be immediately dressed up in Baby's First KKK Hood and given a rattle in the shape of a burning cross).

But. If the patient had a dolphin tattoo on her right groin, would it be so bad if my skin incision was slightly wider than usual and I had no choice but to decapitate the dolphin? I could say, if pushed by an official inquiry (or some Aryan Brotherhood henchman) that I'd been worried the baby was larger than average and it had made sense to have a good-size operative field. And on closing the skin, would it be so bad if the edges of the wound didn't approximate very well for some strange, almost certainly unprovable reason, leaving the dolphin's head positioned a good inch to the left of its body?*

Saturday, May 1, 2010

I'm discussing a case with my colleague Padma in the coffee room after prenatal clinic, and a midwife leaps into the conversation with "We actually don't like to use that word anymore." We wonder what outmoded terminology we've accidentally used (Consumption? Scrofula?), and she lets us know that we said *patient*. We should actually say *client*—calling them patients is paternalistic and demeaning, and pregnancy is a normal and natural process, not a pathological one. I just smile and remember the wise words of Dr. Flitwick, one of my very first consultants, with regards to arguing with midwives—"Do not negotiate with terrorists."

Padma clearly has no such qualms. "I had no idea *patient* was such a demeaning term," she says. "I'm so sorry, I'll never use it again. *Client*. *Client*'s much better. Like what prostitutes have."

---

* Well, we've spoken to a lawyer and the answer, it turns out, is "Yes. That would totally be assault." So we'll say that I didn't do it.

Sunday, May 9, 2010

Having a poo on the labor ward when the emergency buzzer goes off, and within minutes I've delivered a baby at a crash cesarean section. The second the buzzer sounded I crimped it off, but my wiping was cursory, at best, which is why my arse is now unbearably itchy while I'm scrubbed into the OR. It's acceptable to ask someone who's not scrubbed—a midwife or surgical tech—to push your mask or glasses up if they're falling off or even to scratch an itch on your nose. Would it be going too far to ask them for a quick anal scratch?

Monday, May 24, 2010

I never volunteer my opinions on home births, but if, as today, a patient specifically asks me what I think of them, what I'd have if it were me, then I'll be honest. It's a five-minute speech, as follows: I tell them I don't doubt for a second that a home delivery that goes according to plan must be a hundred times more calm, relaxing, and pleasant than a hospital birth. (Though I'm not sure I could ever personally relax knowing that at any moment a blood-and-amniotic-fluid emulsion might slosh onto the sofa. How would you go about getting that out?)

I then tell them I respect patient choice and that it's crucial they feel absolute ownership of their care.

I tell them I get worried by the increasing promotion of "natural" birth and that demedicalization of pregnancy isn't necessarily a good thing—we should be proud of medical advances that objectively save lives, not scared of them.

I say I've seen a number of near misses, including one where we were seconds away from losing a child who'd been transferred to the labor ward when a home birth had gone pear-shaped. I also describe hospital deliveries I've seen in low-risk* mothers where rare and unpredictable events meant they or their babies would certainly have died outside of a hospital.

I promote midwife-based units, where women can have magical, wonderful births in more controlled environments. Crystals, beanbags, someone singing Radiohead songs backward in Swedish—whatever floats your boat, just as long as you're a few hundred yards from a labor ward and its team of shit-fan-separation specialists.

I acknowledge that when it comes to home births I see only the disasters and never the successes, which some people describe as a fatal flaw in my argument. Presumably they also have issues with firefighters who advise the use of seat belts because they see only the victims they angle-grind out of pileups, not the majority of

---

* On booking into antenatal prenatal clinic, patients are categorized as either high or low risk, and low-risk mothers are eligible for home births. People tend to forget that "low risk" doesn't mean "no risk."

people who make safe car journeys. I will put my hand on my heart and tell the patient I implore anyone close to me to think twice about having a home delivery.

Unfortunately, today's clinic is running massively late, and I've got a dinner date, so I don't have time for all this. Instead, I give the abbreviated version: "Home delivery is for pizzas."

Wednesday, June 2, 2010

Teaching medical students this morning—they're keen to brush up on their X-ray-reading skills. I grab a couple of films from the trolley and shove one up on the light box. It's a normal chest X-ray of a patient, taken preoperatively. The first student steps up to present.

"This is a PA chest radiograph taken yesterday of a sixty-four-year-old female patient with name NW and date of birth March first, 1946. There is adequate inspiration and the film is well penetrated and not rotated." He's good.

"The trachea is central, the mediastinum not displaced, and the cardiac contours are normal. The obvious abnormality is a curvilinear mass in the superior lobe of the right lung, occupying—"

Hang on. Abnormality? Where the hell did that come from? Holy fuck. I reviewed this earlier and missed a tumor—I've sent the patient off to surgery and her certain death. I push past the student to get a better look at the cancer. Then I reposition the X-ray slightly and the mass moves. It was a give blood sticker on the light box.*

Saturday, June 5, 2010

My life is starting to feel like an episode of *Quantum Leap*. I'll suddenly wake up and not know where I am or what I have to do. Today, I startle awake to a loud knocking sound—I'm sitting in my car asleep at a set of lights and an old boy is rapping on the window with the handle of his umbrella, asking if I'm okay.

It's the second unexpected power nap of the night shift; earlier, a scrub nurse tapped me on the shoulder while I sat fast asleep on an operating-theater stool to tell me the patient was just being wheeled in for her marsupialization.† We're repeatedly reminded not to

---

*   My friend Percy was working as an orthopedic SHO when there was a trauma call to the ER—a motorcyclist had flown off his bike and broken all sorts of bones. The chest X-ray (routinely performed to check lungs haven't been punctured), Percy was proud to announce, showed varicella pneumonia—a rare and dangerous complication of chicken pox with a characteristic X-ray appearance. The patient was clearly septic with this pneumonia, which caused him to lose control and fly off his bike. Or, as it eventually turned out, his lungs were fine—but loads of gravel had gone up the back of his jacket and shown up on the X-ray.

† Marsupialization is the treatment for a Bartholin's abscess (an infection of the glands that provide vaginal lubrication). You create a pouch to help the abscess drain, hence marsupialization, like a genital kangaroo.

use empty patient rooms to catch any sleep overnight—the management maintains we're paid to work full shifts. I want to ask the management if they've heard of that big ball of fire in the sky that makes it slightly harder to sleep during the day than at night? Or how easy they think it is to suddenly switch from working during the day and sleeping at night to the exact opposite within twenty-four hours? But most of all I want to ask if they or their wives needed an emergency cesarean section at seven a.m., would they rather the registrar doing it had caught forty minutes' sleep when things were quiet or had been forced to stay awake every second of the shift?

It's a surreal feeling being this tired, almost like being in a computer game. You're there but you're not there. I suspect my reaction times are currently the same as when I'm about three pints deep. And yet if I turned up at work drunk, they'd probably be unimpressed—it's clearly important my senses are dulled only through exhaustion.

I left work at 9:30 a.m.—it took me an hour to write up the notes for my last cesarean because I was really struggling to find the words, my tiredness having turned English into a foreign language. Do the courts take this into consideration when you nod off and mow down an entire family on the way home?

Friday, June 11, 2010

I tell a woman in prenatal clinic that she has to give up smoking. She shoots me a look that makes me wonder if I've accidentally just said "I want to fuck your cat" or "They're closing the Dollar Store." She refuses to entertain the idea of a smoking cessation class. I explain how bad smoking is for her baby, but she doesn't particularly seem to care—she tells me all her friends smoked through pregnancy and their kids are fine.

I'm tired and just want to go home. I look at the clock; it's half past six, clinic was meant to end an hour ago and she's far from the last patient on my list. I snap.

"If you don't stop smoking when you're pregnant then nothing on earth will stop you smoking, and you'll die of a smoking-related illness." As I'm saying this I can hear it being repeated back to me slowly by a lawyer—I immediately apologize. But strangely, it seems to have worked—she looks at me like it's the first time she's ever truly listened to anyone, like she's about to stand on the chair and exclaim, "'O Captain! My Captain!'" She doesn't, as luck would have it, because the chair doesn't look like it could take it, but she does ask me about those smoking-cessation classes. Good to know that death threats are effective on my patients.

On her way out she jokes, "Maybe I'll start heroin instead!" I laugh and don't mention that, yes, that would genuinely be safer for her unborn child.

Monday, June 14, 2010

Professor Carrow is the consultant on call for the labor ward today, which is about as much use as having a cardboard cutout of Cher on call for the labor ward. In fact, Cardboard Cher might at least raise morale a bit.

You don't see Professor Carrow during the day, you don't phone him at night—he's far too important for all that nonsense. When he appears on the ward this evening I can only assume that he's got lost or one of his first-degree relatives is currently giving birth.

It all falls into place as a documentary film crew show up behind him, cameras rolling.* "Talk me through the labor-ward board," Carrow says to me, which I do. He nods along for the cameras. "Sounds like you've got it all under control, Adam. But if you've got any problems at all during the night, just call me." The crew have what they want and stop recording. Professor doesn't miss a beat before saying, "Obviously, don't."

---

* In London you're never more than six feet from a rat—and in a big hospital you're never more than six feet from a documentary film crew.

Tuesday, June 15, 2010

I've spent a lot of time with patient VF, as I've been performing FBSs* on her baby every hour. She and her husband have been having a blazing argument for the last four. It started with something about his parents, we've heard all about some friend's wedding where she was flirting with Chris *again*, and now we're on to money. If I were at their dinner party I'd have secreted my uneaten dessert in a napkin, made my excuses, and headed home ages ago, but I don't really have any choice but to eavesdrop. It's a thorough demonstration of the threadbare state of their relationship—I feel like a marriage counselor who's been rendered completely mute.

In truth, they're both behaving equally despicably, but given she's currently in labor—a famously non-fun process—I have to award him 100 percent of the bastard points.

At one stage he goes out to take a phone call and the midwife quite rightly checks with VF that he's not

---

* *Fetal blood sampling (FBS)* is the most accurate way of checking baby's well-being—you lie mum on her side, stick a short length of guttering in her vagina, and make a cut on the top of baby's head using a knife on a long stick. There's no pretending it's any more advanced than this. You then collect a bead of blood in a small tube, and the midwife runs off to drop it, lose it, find that the machine is broken, or, occasionally, report back with the pH of the baby's blood. For some reason they choose not to mention this fairly common procedure in prenatal classes.

been hitting her. She assures the midwife this isn't the case. He returns, the arguments continue, then escalate. He's puce-faced and yelling at her—we all ask him to either calm down or step out of the room. He screams at her, "I never wanted this fucking baby anyway," and storms out, never to reappear in the hospital. Jesus.

Friday, June 18, 2010

Patient RB presented to the ER with an ambulance crew and two police officers. And also, of note, a foot of metal pole protruding from her. She was being chased on foot by the police for some reason or other, and her escape plan involved climbing over some railings into a park. The escape plan unfortunately failed just as she was getting over the railings, when she slipped and one of the metal spikes slid up her vagina and penetrated through the front of her abdomen.

She'd had the presence of mind to get off her face on cocaine earlier in the evening, which anesthetized her sufficiently until the fire brigade arrived on the scene and were able to cut off the railing just below vagina level (while presumably saying "Holy shit" quite a lot). She arrived here hemodynamically stable and remarkably well, all things considered, so we arranged an urgent CT to delineate precisely which cuts of meat were skewered on this particular kebab. Miraculously, she'd avoided damage to her bladder and major blood vessels, so it was just a case of taking her to the operating theater and sewing up the entry and exit wounds.

We evaluated her after surgery—she was sober, sore, embarrassed, and with a police chaperone, as she was still under arrest. We told her that all looked well and gave her a postoperative management plan. She asked if she could keep the spike as a souvenir, and I said I couldn't see any reason why not. The policeman came up with a convincing one—it's really not a good idea to give an arrested criminal a weapon capable of piercing an abdomen.

Tuesday, June 22, 2010

What to do when you're managing an emergency and there's another emergency? I'm on the labor ward when the buzzer goes off—mum's pushing and there's a horrendous-looking trace, baby needs to be urgently lifted out with forceps. I do the necessary and baby comes out quickly, but it's floppy. The pediatrician does her magic and the baby yelps to life. Placenta out and the patient is bleeding moderately from a combination of the generous episiotomy* and a slightly boggy uterus. I'm starting to do part two of the neces-

---

* An *episiotomy* is a cut made with scissors (I'd love to say they were special surgical scissors, but they're just normal scissors) into the perineum to prevent a tear that would be harder to repair or might go into the anus. Essentially, it's a controlled explosion.

sary when I hear another emergency buzzer. I'd bet-ter stay—this could quite easily escalate into a major PPH,* and in any case she's already losing blood every moment I'm not sewing her up or calling out the name of the next drug for the midwife to inject. On the other hand, this other unknown emergency could be much worse, and my current patient is very unlikely to suf-fer permanent harm if I leave her in the hands of an experienced midwife.

It's daytime, but who's to say all my colleagues aren't busy with patients, each assuming someone else will attend the emergency buzzer, which continues to sound. Or what if it's the kind of emergency that needs all hands on deck? I consider sending the midwife to report back, but that minute might be critical for the other patient. I hand the midwife a large swab, tell her to press hard on the perineal wound until I get back, and give her instructions about the next couple of drugs to get into the patient if necessary. I sprint out. The light is flashing outside room three and I bound in, hoping I've made the right decision. Naturally, I haven't.

A midwife is running a CPR drill. There's a man-nequin on the bed and a bunch of doctors and nurses calling out what they'd do were this a real emergency. Which it isn't. Unlike the one I've just left. "Right, the registrar is here," says the midwife to the SHO.

---

* *PPH* means "postpartum hemorrhage" to half of all doctors and "primary pulmonary hypertension" to the other half due to a naming ambiguity.

"What would you like him to do?" What I in fact do is walk up to the mannequin, push it off the bed, call the midwife a cretin, and accuse her of deliberately sabotaging patient safety. Then I bolt back to the first room, where all is thankfully stable, and get my non-imaginary patient as good as new. (Okay, not quite.)

I clearly hadn't expressed my feelings adequately earlier, as the midwife supervisor takes me aside afterward and asks me to apologize to the midwife in question for disrupting her simulation and upsetting her. My apology takes the shape of a clinical-incident form, citing this simulation as a dangerous near miss. I'm sure I used to be nice before this job.

Wednesday, June 23, 2010

An e-mail reminds us of the crucial importance of skills-drill training for all clinical staff. However, before any drill is called, it is now policy to check all rooms to ensure no staff are otherwise engaged in emergencies.

Monday, July 5, 2010

A rare bit of continuity of care today. I saw this patient a month or so back in Dr. Burbage's general gynae clinic, and it sounded very much like she had premature ovarian failure. Early menopause is rather beyond my scope, which I confessed to the patient, then excused myself while I left the room to speak to Dr. Burbage for a management plan. She thought it was beyond her scope too, and it would be best to pop her into Dr. Bryce's specialist endocrinology clinic in the next available slot. The patient wasn't too upset about the waste of her morning, knowing that she was getting to see the expert next time.

Today, however, I'm the registrar in Dr. Bryce's endocrinology clinic, and he's off on holiday. Last time I saw the patient, I said I didn't have the faintest idea about her condition, and now she's sitting opposite me, having given up another afternoon to be here, expecting answers, needing help. Do I say I was just being modest last time? That I've taken a course since then? Do I put on an accent? Fake mustache?

I book her into clinic in a fortnight, when I know I'll be on nights, to avoid the possibility of a hat trick.

Tuesday, July 27, 2010

Ron tried to dump me as a friend today—a proper, somber, grown-up discussion. He doesn't know why he bothers trying to keep in touch with me when it's clear our lives have drifted apart massively since school.

I should at least vary up the excuses I give him. Do I really expect him to believe I couldn't come to his engagement drinks or his bachelor party because of work? That I couldn't make the wedding ceremony because of work and almost missed the reception as well? That I missed his dad's funeral and his daughter's christening because of work? He knows my job's full-on, but how hard can it be to swap shifts if it's something you really want to do?

I put my hand on my heart and swear to Ron that I love him, he's one of my best friends, and I wouldn't lie to him. I know I've been useless, but I've seen a lot more of him than almost anyone else I know—the job is just unimaginably busy. Nonmedical types can never appreciate quite how tough it is to be a doctor and the impact it has on real life. I totally lied about the christening, though—fuck that shit.

Monday, August 2, 2010

It's the final shift of the job—a night shift, naturally. My new post starts an hour before this one ends, about ten miles away, but I'll cross that bridge when I come to it, two hours late and bleary-eyed.

Technically this job ended at midnight, a fact that occurs to me on the stairwell at 12:10 a.m. when my swipe card refuses to let me back onto the ward and I realize it's been automatically deactivated. I'm Cinderella in scrubs.

If you ask the hospital to adequately staff a department, provide an effective computer system, or even supply enough chairs for clinic, you'll get a shrug and a display of colossal incompetence. And yet when it comes to being able to get in and out of doors, it some-how takes on the organizational skills of a cyborg librarian. If swipe cards suddenly start developing cancer, a cure will be found immediately.

I endure a mere quarter of an hour of banging on doors and praying the crash bleeper doesn't go off before someone spots me and lets me back onto the ward.*

---

* The savvy obstetrician doesn't carry his mobile phone in his scrubs. All it takes is one iPhone drowning in a tsunami of blood for you to learn your lesson, and I can assure you that no amount of drying it in rice will revive it.

9

Senior Registrar

Medicine is the host who manages to keep you at the party hours after you first think about leaving. "Don't go before we've cut the birthday cake . . . You must meet Steve before you head off . . . I think Julie lives over your way—she's off home in a minute, why don't you go together . . ." Then before you know it, you've missed the last train back and you're crashing on the sofa.

Having gone to medical school, you might as well finish and become a house officer, then you might as well become an SHO, then you might as well become a registrar, then you might as well become a senior registrar, and by then you're practically a consultant. There almost certainly don't need to be so many different grades; I strongly suspect it's designed so that the next step is always just round the corner. It's the fifty-pound note you chase down the street, swept up by another gust of wind the millisecond before your hand makes contact. And it definitely works. One day I realized—as if blinking awake after a serious accident—that I was now in my thirties and still in a career I'd signed up for fourteen years earlier based on the very flimsiest of reasons.

My ID card and salary now proudly said *Senior registrar* (although in fairness, my salary also said *Bank teller* or *Reasonably experienced milkman*), and my next few postings would bridge the gap from junior doctor to consultant. And, in fact, life as a consultant looked pretty appealing. The pay went up, the hours went down. Admin sessions, days off. No one forcing me to do urogynae clinics. My name in capital letters at the top of my parents' will (probably followed by *He's a consultant gynecologist, you know*). And, best of all, stability: a job that I could stay in as long as I wanted, one where I didn't have to pack my bags as soon as I'd memorized the code on the changing-room door.

But first I had to get through my senior registrar posts—the storm before the calm. Yes, my registrar jobs had been manic and relentless, but this was a different kind of stress—now I was the highest-ranking person in the department after hours. Knowing that when my bleeper went off, it was a problem that both the SHO and the registrar had failed to resolve. Knowing that if I couldn't deal with it, a mother or a baby might die. Having consultants at home on call was just a formality; most emergencies were over in a matter of minutes, before they could even change out of their dressing gowns. I would now need to accept ultimate responsibility for the fails and fuckups of an SHO and registrar I might have never met before. While I'd often go unbleeped for an hour or two on a night shift, I preferred to prowl anxiously around the labor ward, flitting from room to room asking, "Is everything okay?," suffering the occasional flashback to that registrar who told me as a student that obs and gynae was an easy specialty. Lying bastard.

So it wasn't the biggest surprise in the world when I saw a GP and the practice nurse recorded my blood pressure as 182/108 mm Hg.* She wouldn't accept my explanation that I was just off a night shift with two locums, still tightly wound from twelve hours on the wards, my mind jittering with a dozen medical equivalents of "Did I turn the gas off?" Did the patient have that CT scan? Did I put in a second layer of stitches? Did I prescribe that methotrexate?

She booked me back in to see the GP the following week, and my pressure was just as high. Again, I was straight back from work. I assured her I'd checked my BP myself in clinic and it was completely normal, but she wanted to be sure just the same. In fairness to her, I

---

* You want your blood pressure to be under 120/80 mm Hg (aka millimeters of mercury). If you stuck a glass tube full of mercury into your heart, it's the number of millimeters the pressure would push the level up—though these days we use a slightly less invasive method to measure it. The top number is the pressure when your heart is going *lub*; the bottom number is when it's going *dub*.

was totally lying; I'd done no such thing. She arranged for me to have twenty-four-hour ambulatory monitoring.* Because days off work were in short supply, I wore it on a prenatal clinic day, making it practicable (I wouldn't have to go to the OR) plus theoretically low stress. I sat in clinic and explained to patients that I needed to start them on antihypertensive medication, despite the device strapped to my arm proudly displaying that my blood pressure was significantly higher than theirs.

Among all the predictably "hilarious" remarks the patients made to me, one said something surprisingly astute. "It's funny—you don't think of doctors getting ill." It's true, and I think it's part of something bigger: patients don't actually think of doctors as being human. It's why they're so quick to complain if we make a mistake or if we get cross. It's why they'll bite our heads off when we finally call them into our over-running clinic room at seven p.m., not thinking that we also have homes we'd rather be at. But it's the flip side of not wanting your doctor to be fallible, capable of getting your diagnosis wrong. They don't want to think of medicine as a subject that anyone on the planet

---

* _Ambulatory monitoring_ involves wandering round for a day with a blood-pressure cuff on your arm that inflates every fifteen minutes or so and records the data for the doctor. It's particularly useful in "white-coat hypertension," when patients get nervous and their blood pressure rockets up. About a week before finals at medical school, my friend Antonin asked during a tutorial, "Why's it called white-goat hypertension?" He's a consultant hematologist now if you want to watch out for him.

can learn, a career choice their mouth-breathing cousins could have made.

After an hour at home, my blood pressure returned to normal, so mercifully my arteries were still in decent shape. Plus it was interesting to be able to quantify in millimeters of mercury precisely how stressful it was to be a senior registrar.

Monday, August 9, 2010

A patient named her baby after me today. It was a planned cesarean for a breech presentation, and after I delivered the baby I said, "Adam's a good name." The parents agreed, and the deal's done.

I say, "Adam's a good name," after every single baby I deliver, and this was the first time that anyone's ever said yes. I've not even had it used as a middle name before. But today this wrong was righted, and the squad of Adams I so richly deserve was launched in OR two. (I'm not sure what I'll do with this team once they're assembled. Fight crime, maybe? Get them to cover my shifts?)

The SHO assisting me in the cesarean asked how many babies I'd delivered. I estimated twelve hundred. He then looked up some population data and told me that, on average, nine of every twelve hundred babies born in the UK would be called Adam. I have genuinely put eight sets of parents off naming their child after me.

Sunday, August 15, 2010

Summoned to a delivery room by one of the junior registrars—she's struggling to lock a pair of forceps onto the baby's head. We've had the occasional set of mismatched pairs sent to us recently—two left sides or slightly different models packed together after sterilization. On examination, the left blade is placed well on the side of baby's head. The right blade, however, is wedged halfway up the patient's rectum.

Mistake corrected and baby delivered safely. (By me—at this point, I wouldn't trust the registrar to deliver a limerick.)

"Do we have to tell her?" she asks conspiratorially, testing my ethical boundaries like I'm a builder and she's hoping to pay in cash and avoid the tax.

"Of course not," I say. "*You* do."

Monday, August 23, 2010

Week three of the job and I'm just about up to speed with the eligibility criteria for infertility* treatment here. Today I saw a couple who've had an unsuccessful round of IVF, which was unsurprising. Chances of

---

* *Infertility clinic* got rebranded to "subfertility clinic" during the course of my training to make it sound less negative, then again to "fertility clinic," which feels a bit "La-la-la, this isn't happening" fingers-in-ears-y. Unless over in oncology they're now running the "Definitely not got breast cancer" clinic?

success in their particular case were around 20 percent for a single cycle. Where I worked a month ago, a walkable distance away, they'd have qualified for three cycles, which would have upped their odds to nearer 50 percent. They ask me what private treatment would cost and I tell them: around four thousand pounds for a cycle. The look on their faces tells me I may as well have said four trillion pounds.*

People say it's a choice to have kids, which is of course true. But no one argues that patients with recurrent miscarriages shouldn't be allowed treatment until they have a baby—and the NHS rightly doesn't limit their care. And how about the patient who had two ectopic pregnancies, leaving her with no fallopian tubes and no chance of getting pregnant without IVF? All we're doing is allowing people to make a choice they would have otherwise had were it not for a medical condition. Or not, because their surname begins

---

* In most aspects of private medicine, you get a mild upgrade on the NHS but no huge difference in actual care. You get seen a bit quicker, the receptionist's got all her teeth, and there's a decent wine list for your inpatient stay, but ultimately you get the same treatment. When it comes to infertility medicine, though, the private sector is leagues ahead; they will investigate and treat you until you have a baby (or declare bankruptcy). The NHS requires you to fit into quite a narrow demographic to qualify for any treatment, and it's often not enough to achieve a positive result. I understand there's a limited pot of money, but you don't ever hear this said in other corners of medicine. "We don't treat leukemia—there's a limited pot of money." "We only treat fractures on the right side of the body—there's a limited pot of money."

with the letter G. I'm exaggerating, of course—that would be ridiculous. They'd only be denied it for sensible reasons, such as living one road outside of an arbitrary catchment area.

I suggest they take a bit of a break to think about their options and come to terms with their feelings. I float the possibilities of fostering or adoption. "It's not the same, though, is it?" the husband says, and no, it's probably not.

In the short time I've been working here I've told a lesbian couple they are eligible for treatment but a gay male couple wanting surrogacy that they're not. I've told a woman she's too old for treatment according to our criteria, even though she wasn't too old when she was referred here a few months ago. (And wouldn't have been too old a few streets away.) I've been cast in the role of a malevolent god.

Here there's a BMI limit for receiving treatment, something I've never encountered before. I had to tell a patient she was three kilos too heavy to be referred for IVF and to see me again when she'd lost the weight. She burst into tears, so I accidentally recorded her weight on the form as a few kilos too light.* Last week I wrote a letter citing exceptional circumstances, requesting treatment be allowed for a woman who had a child from a previous relationship who'd died in infancy, which cruelly makes her ineligible for treatment here.

---

* Is this the "One weird weight-loss trick that doctors don't want you to know about" much vaunted by internet ads?

I leave clinic, passing a rack of leaflets that details all the different fertility treatment options that the NHS in this area makes it all but impossible to receive. We should be more honest and replace them all with one titled "Have You Thought About Getting a Cat?"

Wednesday, August 25, 2010

An eighty-five-year-old, long-stay gynae-oncology patient broke our hearts on yesterday's ward rounds. She misses her late husband, her children have barely visited since she's been in hospital, and she can't even have her usual whiskey nightcap in here. I decided to play Boy Scout, prescribed whiskey (fifty milliliters nightly) on her drug chart, and gave the house officer twenty pounds to get a bottle from the supermarket to pass on to the nursing staff so they could deliver the medication on their drug round.

This morning, the charge nurse reports that the patient declined her drink because, and I quote: "Jack Daniel's is fucking cat piss."

Monday, September 13, 2010

A new midwife supervisor, Tracy, has started this week and seems absolutely lovely—calm, experienced, and sensible. She is now the second midwife supervisor on the unit called Tracy, the current one being a flappy, angry nightmare. To avoid confusion, we have nicknamed them "Reassuring Trace" and "Non-Reassuring Trace."

Friday, September 24, 2010

Moral maze. It's Friday, it's five to five, it's a bleep from the OR staff with something enormously time-consuming. There's a patient with an ectopic pregnancy needing emergency surgery, and they would like me to pop up now. This is particularly annoying timing, as it's date night. In fact, it's more than date night. It's date night somewhere extremely expensive to apologize for half a dozen recently canceled date nights and to paper over the widening fault lines in our relationship. It's D-date night. I should be fine if I leave by 6:00 p.m., I tell myself. At 5:45 it's time to start operating. The evening registrar is stuck in the ER and can't relieve me.

Best practice is to operate laparoscopically—about an hour's work for me, it leaves the patient with a couple of tiny holes, and she'll be home tomorrow. Alternatively, I can make a quick incision in this twenty-five-year-old's pristine abdomen and sentence her to a proper scar and a longer hospital stay but get away on time and keep my relationship on track. Besides, maybe the patient likes hospital food? I hesitate for a moment more, then request the laparoscopy set.

Tuesday, October 5, 2010

On the phone to my friend Sophia, having a moan about the levels of exhaustion and demoralization in our hospitals. We're both pretty fed up. She tells me she's just got her private pilot's license and is planning to take a break from the NHS. "And work for an airline?" I ask.

Actually, she's going to charter an aircraft and fly it around twenty-four African countries, visiting remote areas where maternal morbidity is the highest and teaching the local midwives some lifesaving techniques. She'll also donate huge amounts of medical supplies and educational resources which she's going to fund-raise for before she sets off. Now I feel exhausted, demoralized, and selfish.

Monday, October 11, 2010

A text out of the blue from Simon; no news has been good news for the last eighteen months, so my heart rather sinks when I see his name pop up. He's just asking for my address—he wants to send me a wedding invitation. I'm choked up that he'd think of me and very much looking forward to intending to go, then pulling out at the last minute due to work.

Tuesday, October 12, 2010

The final patient of a comically busy prenatal clinic requests an elective cesarean section because of a previous traumatic vaginal delivery. This is a fairly common request—principally because there's no such thing as a nontraumatic vaginal delivery. The SHO who saw her previously did the sensible thing and requested the notes from the hospital where she had her last baby, and I skim through them to see if anything particularly traumatizing had happened.

She had a long labor, resulting in a forceps extraction, and needed repair in the OR afterward for a cervical tear. That night, she had a gargantuan postpartum hemorrhage, which caused her to arrest. She was successfully resuscitated—clearly, given she's sitting in clinic—and was taken back to the OR to resew her tear. This second attempt—almost unbelievably—went even worse and resulted in damage to her small bowel and, ultimately, to a small-bowel resection and stoma formation. Then a series of clinic letters from psychiatry, documenting her gradual recovery from PTSD caused by these events and the collapse of her marriage. And now she's back to do it again. The woman must be so hard you can skate on her; let her have what she wants.

I book her for an elective section. It's nice to have the bar set so low that almost anything we do will be a considerable upgrade on the last time.

Thursday, October 14, 2010

I was slightly weirded out the first time a patient started texting during an internal examination, but now it seems reasonably common. Today, during a pap smear, a patient FaceTimed her friend.

Sunday, October 17, 2010

I answer an emergency buzzer late at night—it's a shoulder dystocia.*

It's clearly a big baby, quadruple-chinned through how tightly its neck is being squeezed back against mum's perineum, and it's an experienced midwife, someone I know will have already tried everything in the book. There's no pretending to the patient this isn't serious, but she's a dream so far—remaining calm and going along with everything asked of her.

I drain the bladder with a catheter, put her legs in the McRoberts position, apply suprapubic pressure.

---

* *Shoulder dystocia* is one of the scariest experiences for an obstetrician—the baby's head delivers, but the shoulders get stuck. All the time this is going on, baby's brain isn't getting any oxygen, so it's a ticking time bomb of a matter of minutes before irreversible brain damage occurs. We all train regularly in how to manage this particular emergency. Embedded into our brain stems are all manner of mnemonics to help us through it, and all sorts of physical maneuvers: exerting suprapubic pressure, McRoberts (hyperflexing the legs), Wood's screw (rotating the baby by its shoulders), delivering the posterior arm.

This is like no shoulder dystocia I've dealt with before. There's no give at all; the baby isn't budging. I ask the midwife supervisor to see if there are somehow any obstetric consultants in the building. I attempt the Wood's screw maneuver—nothing. I attempt to deliver the posterior arm—impossible. I roll the patient onto all fours and try all the maneuvers again in this position. I ask the midwife to get my consultant on the phone. It's approaching five minutes of shoulder dystocia and something needs to happen urgently if the baby's going to live.

As I see it, I have three options as last-ditch attempts. The first is Zavanelli's maneuver—push the baby's head back inside and perform a crash cesarean section. I've never seen it done but I'm confident I can manage it. I'm also fairly confident that by the time we get her delivered in the OR, the baby will have died.

Second option is to intentionally fracture baby's clavicle to allow baby to deliver. I have never seen this done either and have no real idea how to go about it—it's a famously difficult procedure, even in much better hands than mine.

Third option is to perform a symphysiotomy, cutting the mother's pubic bone to make the outlet bigger. Again, I've never seen it performed, but I'm sure I can do it easily and that it will be the quickest way to get the baby out. I inform the consultant over the phone that this is what I'm going to do—she checks what I've tried so far and confirms my understanding of how to perform it. She's driving in from home, but we both know that by the time she arrives everything will be over, one way or the other.

I feel as sick as I've ever felt in a clinical situation; I'm about to break a patient's pelvis and it might already be too late for her baby. Before I take the scalpel to her I have one last attempt to deliver the baby's posterior arm. All the various maneuvers and shifts in position have somehow made something budge, and the arm delivers, followed by a very limp baby, who the midwife passes to the pediatricians. As we wait for the cry that may or may not come, I remember an old phrase in the textbooks that describes a successful shoulder-dystocia delivery as due to "greater strength of muscle or by some infernal juggle" and totally get what the author was on about. The baby cries. Hallelujah. The midwife bursts into tears. We will have to wait and see if there's an Erb's,* but the pediatrician whispers in my ear that both arms seem to be behaving normally.

I see that I've given the mother a third-degree tear, which isn't ideal but is pretty minor collateral damage in the grand scheme of things. I ask the midwife to prepare her for the OR—that'll give me twenty minutes to write up my delivery notes and grab a cup of coffee. My SHO comes in—can I quickly do a vacuum extraction in another room?

---

* *Erb's palsy* is nerve damage to the arm resulting from straining the neck in this kind of scenario.

Wednesday, October 20, 2010

Maybe it's because his first language is Greek. Maybe he's forgotten our previous discussion where I'd offered to help him with ultrasound technique. Maybe I should have phrased it as "determine fetal gender." But judging by the SHO's look of confusion and disgust and his hasty retreat down the corridor, what I shouldn't have said was a cheery "Would you like to watch me sex a baby?"

Thursday, October 21, 2010

I pick up notes for the next patient I'm seeing in gynae clinic. I recognize the name; flicking through the notes, I see a clinic letter I wrote to her GP back in March. I spot a horrifying typo in my sign-off, thanks to a missing *hesitate to.*

If you have any questions whatsoever, please do not contact me.

It worked, though. Not a peep.

Wednesday, October 27, 2010

I'm in occupational health for a follow-up HIV test after a needlestick injury from a positive patient three months ago. She had an undetectable viral load but it's still not ideal by any stretch, and I've had it constantly in the back of my mind since, like a tax bill.

Making nervous small talk with the occupational-health registrar as he takes my blood, I ask what happens to an obstetrician who's HIV positive. "You wouldn't be able to do clinical procedures, so no labor ward, OR, on-calls—just clinics, I guess." I don't say it, but that would really take the sting out of the diagnosis.*

Sunday, October 31, 2010

At a friend's Halloween party I spot someone I know from somewhere. School, I think.

I amble over to say hi. Blank face. Not school. University? Nope.

Where did you grow up? Have we worked together? Humiliatingly for me, but probably for his own sanity, he has to stop me and say that I've probably just seen him on TV—he's a television personality, called Danny. Humiliatingly for *him*, I say the name maybe rings a bell, but I'm pretty sure that's not it. His wife

---

* Since 2013, it's been okay for an HIV-positive doctor with an undetectable viral load to operate, after a decade of lobbying that the risk to patients was negligible. My blood test was negative, in case you wondered whether the book was about to take a dark turn.

wanders over and I work it out—I delivered their baby by cesarean a year or so back.

Much hugging, hand-shaking, and what-a-coincidence-ing. Danny jokes he's glad it was a cesarean, because he doesn't know how he'd feel about talking to a man who's seen his wife's vagina. I want to say that *actually* I'd have seen it when catheterizing her for the procedure, plus, if he really wants something to get his brain imploding, I'd also have seen its reverse side during the operation. I don't say this, just in case he wasn't joking and things get even more awkward.

Monday, November 8, 2010

The cherry on top of a record-breakingly hellish night shift (with a locum registrar who was of barely more than ornamental value) is a crash cesarean at 7:45 a.m., fifteen minutes from the supposed finish line. Cesarean, then another cesarean, then vacuum extraction, then forceps, then cesarean, then I lost count, but a bunch more babies, and now a final cesarean. I'm absolutely exhausted and would gladly have dragged my feet and handed this C-section over to the morning shift were the trace not preterminal.*

I've not sat down for twelve hours, let alone rested my eyes, my dinner's sitting uneaten in my locker, and

---

* *Preterminal* means the baby will die if nothing is done.

I've just called a midwife "Mum" by accident. We run to the OR and I deliver the baby very quickly—it's limp, but the pediatricians do their black magic and soon it's making the right sort of noises. Cord gases confirm we made the right decision and I close up the patient on a vague high.

The pediatrician grabs me for a word after I leave the operating theater and tells me I've cut the baby's cheek with my scalpel while making the uterine incision—it's not bad, but just to let me know. I go straight to see the baby and parents. It's not a deep cut, nor is it long—it didn't need any skin closure and it surely won't scar—but it was totally my fault. I apologize to the parents, who couldn't seem to give less of a toss. They're in love with their gorgeous (and only mildly mutilated) little girl, and they tell me they understand she had to be delivered in a bit of a rush—these things happen. I want to say that these things aren't meant to happen, that they haven't happened to me before, and they almost certainly wouldn't have happened to me at the start of the shift.

I offer them a leaflet with the details of the hospital's complaints procedure—they don't want it. A close shave for my GMC registration and an actual shave for the poor baby. A couple of centimeters higher and I'd have taken her eye out, a couple of millimeters deeper and I could have caused scarring and blood loss. Babies have even died from lacerations at cesarean. I document our discussion in the notes, fill in the clinical-incident form, do everything demanded of me by the system that allowed this to happen in the first place. Before long I'll get sat down by someone to be gently or not-so-gently chastised, and at no point will it occur to this person that there might be a more fundamental problem here.*

Thursday, November 11, 2010

I suspected the husband of the couple in infertility clinic had a urinary tract infection so I gave him a specimen cup and sent him off to the restroom for a sample. He peered at it for a few seconds before tottering off. I suppose it was my fault for not being specific enough, but he returned (admirably quickly) with the pot containing a few milliliters of semen. The miscommunication could have been worse, of course—he could've shat in it, bled into it, or stuck a skewer into the ventricles of his brain to draw out a cup of cerebrospinal fluid. I do rather wonder whether the reason they're struggling to conceive is that he's urinating into his wife during sex.

---

* Almost a decade previously, I worked at the same hospital as a medical secretary during university holidays. We were obliged to take a twenty-minute break after every two hours of staring at a computer screen because of "health and safety."

Sunday, November 14, 2010

It's Sunday lunchtime and patient RZ needs a cesarean section for failure to progress in labor. The patient is happy to have a section, but her husband doesn't want me to perform it because I'm male. They are ortho-dox Muslims and have apparently been told they can have all female doctors. I say I don't know who told them that but, although there are often women doc-tors available, we work on a schedule and currently the entire team in obs and gynae is male, including the consultant on call at home.

"So you're honestly telling me that there are no fe-male doctors in the hospital?"

"No, sir, I'm telling you there are no female doctors in the hospital capable of performing a cesarean. I'm sure I could easily find your wife a female dermatolo-gist."

The patient is clearly much happier with the idea of me doing the section than her husband is, but she's not really being allowed to speak up. We go through the motions, getting even further away from the re-sult we need the more we dance around it. "When's a woman doctor next here?" When the shifts change in seven hours, which would be a very bad idea for your baby. "Can't the midwife do it?" No, and neither can housekeeping.

I call the consultant for some moral support. He sug-gests I get in drag, and I suspect he's only half joking. Back in the room, I ask, "Does the Koran not allow for male doctors to operate in the case of an emergency?" Which, I remind them, this is. It's a total bluff, but it seems the sort of thing a religious text might say. They ask me to give them five minutes, make some phone calls, then the husband comes to find me to say that they're happy for me to deliver the baby. He says it in a way that implies I should be grateful. In fact, I am grateful, but only because my main concern was the safe appearance of his child, not his (or anyone else's) God's feelings on the matter. Plus I don't have a plan B and can't begin to contemplate the unending quantity of paperwork that would otherwise haunt me forever.

Before long we're in the OR, and I've safely delivered their baby girl. Healthy mum, healthy baby—it's all we ever aim for, and they should be glad everything worked out fine for them when it doesn't for so many families who come through these doors.

In the event, the husband is extremely thankful—he apologizes for wasting my time and adding to my stress and tells me he's grateful for all I've done. As with most husbands who go off on us, he was probably just stressed by the situation, and I presume the added jeopardy of potential eternal damnation didn't help either.

He's going down to the shops; would I like anything? I half want to see his reaction if I ask for a BLT, a bottle of Smirnoff, and some poppers.

Thursday, November 18, 2010

Was meant to be back home at 7:00 p.m. sharp but it's 9:30 and I've only just come off the labor ward. Feels appropriate that work commitments mean I have to reschedule collecting all my belongings from the flat. On the plus side, my depressing new bachelor pad is only ten minutes from the hospital.

Monday, November 22, 2010

A patient awaiting evaluation in the ER for some minor abdominal pain has sunk lower and lower down my list of priorities throughout the afternoon as the labor ward has become busier and busier. I'm in the middle of stabilizing a patient with severe preeclampsia when I'm bleeped by a furious ER registrar.

"If you don't come to the ER right now, this patient is going to breach the four-hour target."*

"Okay. But if I *do* come right now, my current patient is going to die." Mic drop.

There's a good five seconds of radio silence during which he clearly wonders if there's anything he can

---

* Because hospitals aren't under quite enough pressure, the government has decided that all patients in the ER need to be admitted or discharged within four hours, whether they've had strokes or stubbed their toes. If more than 5 percent of these patients breach the target (unfortunately not the type of breech that interests me), the hospital gets fined and the management unleashes a heap of hell on the ER staff.

fire back that will persuade me to come down and save him a load of aggro. I spend this time marveling at a system that's so obsessed with arbitrary targets that his reply should take this long to generate.

"Fine. Just come when you can," he replies. "But I'm really not happy about this." When my pre-eclamptic patient is out of the woods, I must remember to have her write him an apology.

Friday, November 26, 2010

The last of my preoperative patients I have to consent before the OR is QS, an elderly lady having a hysteroscopy following some recent PV bleeding. She's accompanied by a corduroy-wearing trust-fund douche of a son. He's under the impression that the more he treats the medical staff like crap, the more convinced they will be of his importance, and thus the better treatment his family will receive. Amazingly, this is a commonly held belief, and annoyingly, he's absolutely right. This is the type who would complain to the management if his mother got so much as a chip in her toenail polish.

I bite my tongue harder with every question he asks. "How many of these have you done?" "Is this not a case that your consultant should be doing?" If this were a restaurant and I were a waiter, I would currently be stirring my spit and semen into his beef bourguignon, but she's a sweet old lady, and she's not going to suffer just because her son's an arsehole. We're all done.

"Treat her as if she's your own mother," he instructs me. I assure him he really doesn't want *that* at all.

Sunday, December 5, 2010

Spending my Sunday afternoon on the labor ward with an excellent SHO. She asks me to evaluate a CTG and I agree with her assessment that the patient needs a cesarean section for fetal distress. They are a lovely couple, recently married; it's their first baby, and they understand the situation.

The SHO asks if she can perform the cesarean while I assist. In the operating theater, the SHO goes through the layers: skin, fat, muscles, peritoneum one, peritoneum two, uterus. After the uterine incision, rather than amniotic fluid, blood comes out—lots of blood. There has been an abruption.* I stay calm and ask the SHO to deliver the baby—she says she can't, there's something in the way. I take over the operation—the placenta is in the way. The patient has an undiagnosed placenta previa. This should have been noticed on scans; she should never have been allowed to go into labor. I deliver the placenta and then deliver the baby. The baby is clearly dead. Pediatricians attempt resuscitation but without success.

---

* *Abruption* is a complication of pregnancy where all or part of the placenta separates from the uterus. Because all of baby's oxygen and nutrients are delivered via the placenta, this can be extremely serious indeed.

The patient is bleeding heavily from the uterus—one liter, two liters. My sutures have no effect, drugs have no effect. I call for the consultant to come in urgently. The patient is now under general anesthesia and receiving emergency blood transfusions; her husband has been escorted out of the theater. Blood loss is now five liters. I try a brace suture*—no luck. I'm squeezing the uterus as hard as I can with both hands—it's the only thing that stops the bleeding.

The consultant arrives, attempts another brace suture; it doesn't work. I see the panic in her eyes. The anesthesiologist tells us he can't get fluid into the patient fast enough to replace what she's losing and we're risking organ damage. The consultant calls another colleague—he's not on duty, but he's the most experienced surgeon she can think of. We take it in turns squeezing the uterus until he arrives twenty minutes later. He performs a hysterectomy; the bleeding is finally under control. Twelve liters. The patient goes to intensive care and I am warned to expect the worst. My consultant talks to the husband. I start to write up my operation notes but instead just cry for an hour.

---

* *Brace sutures* are very large stitches that go around the uterus like a pair of braces to compress it and stop the bleeding.

10

Aftermath

That was the last diary entry I wrote, and the reason there aren't any more laughs in this book.

Everyone at the hospital was very kind to me and said all the right things; they told me it wasn't my fault, said I couldn't have done anything differently, and sent me home for the rest of the shift. And yet at the same time, it felt a bit like I'd sprained my ankle. A flurry of people asking me "Are you okay?" but also the definite expectation that I'd still come into work the next day, the reset button firmly pressed. That's not to say they were heartless or unthinking—it's a problem that's baked into the profession. You can't wear a black armband every time something goes wrong; you can't take a month's compassionate leave—it happens too often.

It's a system that barely has enough slack to allow for sick leave, let alone something as intangible as recovering from an awful day. And, in truth, doctors *can't* acknowledge how devastating these moments really are. If you're going to survive working in this profession, you have to convince yourself these horrors are just part of your job. You can't pay any attention to the man behind the curtain—your own sanity relies on it.

I'd seen babies die before. I'd dealt with mothers on the brink of death before. But this was different. It was the first time I was the most senior person on the ward when something terrible happened, when I was the person everyone was relying on to sort it all out. It was on me, and I had failed.

Officially, I hadn't been negligent and nobody suggested otherwise. Medical negligence will always be judged by asking the question "Would your peers have done anything differently in that situation?" All my peers would have done exactly the same things and had exactly the same outcome. But this wasn't good enough for me. I knew that if I'd been better—super-diligent, super-observant, super-something—I might have gone into that room an hour earlier. I might have noticed some subtle changes on the CTG. I might have saved the baby's life, saved the mother from permanent compromise. That "might have" was inescapable.

Yes, I went back to work the next day. I was in the same skin, but I was a different doctor—I couldn't risk anything bad ever happening again. If a baby's heart rate dropped by one beat per minute, I would perform a cesarean. And it would be me doing it, no SHOs or junior registrars. I knew women were having unnecessary cesareans and I knew colleagues were missing opportunities to improve their surgical skills, but if it meant everyone got out of there alive, it was worth it. I'd mocked consultants for being overcautious before, rolled my eyes the moment they turned their heads, but now I got it. They'd each had their own "might have" moment, and this is how you dealt with it.

Except I wasn't *really* dealing with it, I was just getting on with it. I went six months without laughing; every smile was just an impression of one—I felt bereaved. I should have had counseling—in fact, my hospital should have arranged it. But there's a mutual code of silence that keeps help from those who need it most.

No matter how vigilant I was, another tragedy would have happened eventually. It has to—you can't prevent the unpreventable. One brilliant consultant tells her trainees that by the time they retire, there'll be a bus full of dead kids and kids with cerebral palsy, and that bus is going to have their name on its side. A huge number of "adverse outcomes," as they say in hospital-ese, will occur on their watch. She tells them if they can't deal with that, they're in the wrong profession. Maybe if someone had said that to me a bit earlier, I'd have thought twice. Ideally, back when I was choosing my A levels and getting myself into this mess.

I asked if I could go part-time ("Not unless you're pregnant") and investigated switching to general practice. But first I'd have to drop right down to SHO grade for a couple of years to work in emergency medicine, pediatrics, and psychiatry. I didn't want to take a long journey backward in order to start moving forward again only to find I didn't like that either.

I paused my training with the deanery and did some half-hearted research and lazy locum shifts on private units, but after a few months I hung up my stethoscope. I was done.

I didn't tell anyone the reason why I left. Maybe I should have; maybe they'd have understood. My parents reacted like I'd told them I was being tried for arson. At first I *couldn't* talk about it, then it became something I just *didn't* talk about. When cornered, I would reach for my red nose and clown horn and bring out my anecdotes about objects in anuses and patients "saying the funniest things." Some of my closest friends will read this book and hear this story for the first time.

These days, the only doctoring I do is on other people's words—I write and script-edit comedy for television. A bad day at work now is if my laptop crashes or a terrible sitcom gets terrible ratings—stuff that literally doesn't matter in the scheme of things. I don't miss the doctor's version of a bad day, but I do miss the good days. I miss my colleagues and I miss helping people. I miss that feeling on the drive home that you've done something worthwhile. And I feel guilty the country spent so much money training me for me just to walk away.

I still have a very strong affinity with the profession—

you never totally stop being a doctor. You still run to the injured cyclist sprawled across the road; you still reply to the text messages from friends of friends looking for free fertility advice. So in 2016, when the government started waging war on doctors—forcing them to work harder than ever for less money than ever—I felt huge solidarity with them. And when our government repeatedly lied that doctors were simply being greedy, that they were in medicine for the money—for anything other than the best interests of the patient—I was livid. Because I knew it wasn't true.

The junior doctors lost that particular battle, largely because the government's booming, baleful voice drowned out their own reasonable, experienced quiet one. I realized that every health-care professional—every single doctor, nurse, midwife, pharmacist, physical therapist, and paramedic—needs to shout about the reality of their work so the next time the health secretary lies that doctors are in it for the money, the public will know just how ridiculous that is. Why would any sane person do that job for anything other than the right reasons? Because I wouldn't wish it on anyone. I have so much respect for those who work on the front line because, when it came down to it, I certainly couldn't.

Putting this book together, six years after quitting medicine, I met up with dozens of former colleagues. Their dispatches from the labor ward tell of an NHS on its knees. Every one of them spoke of an exodus from medicine. When I left, I was a glitch in the matrix, an aberration. Now every schedule bears the scars of doctors who've activated their plan Bs—working in Canada or Australia, in pharmaceutical companies or in investment banks. Most of my old colleagues were themselves desperately groping for a ripcord to parachute out of the profession—brilliant, passionate doctors who've had their reasons to stay bullied out of them by politicians. Once upon a time, these people were rescheduling their own weddings for this job.

The other recurrent theme, doctor after doctor, is how they remember the sad stuff, the bad stuff, so vividly. Your brain presses Record in HD. They can tell you the number of the room it happened in on a labor ward they last saw a decade ago. The shoes the patient's husband was wearing, the song playing on the radio. Senior consultants' voices shake when they talk about their disasters—six-foot-tall former rugby champions on the verge of tears. A friend told me about a perimortem cesarean he performed: A mum dropped dead in front of him and he cut the baby out on the floor. It survived. "You saved the wrong one! You saved the wrong one!" was all the dad could cry.

I'm not the right person to talk about dealing with grief, though—that's not what this book is about. It's simply one doctor's experiences, some degree of insight on an individual level into what the job really entails.

But promise me this. Next time a government tries to denigrate doctors or take a pickax to the healthcare system, don't just accept what the politicians feed

you. Think about the toll the job takes on every medical professional, at home and at work. Remember that
all of them do an absolutely impossible job to the very
best of their abilities. Your time in the hospital may
well hurt them a lot more than it hurts you.

ACKNOWLEDGMENTS

With love and thanks to Jess Cooper and Cath Summerhayes at Curtis Brown. Jess, I'm sorry you had to read it so many times while heavily pregnant. To Francesca Main, my most incredible editor—I don't have the words. As usual.

To James, my copilot throughout.

To Drs. Kay, Kay, Kay, and Kay. Sophie—you'll be a much better obstetrician than I was. And Dan, you made the right choice by rebelling (and studying law). To my parents, Naomi and Stewart—love you, really.

To everyone at Picador, particularly Ami Smithson, Dusty Miller, Paul Martinovic, Tom Noble, Paul Baggaley, Kish Widyaratna, Christine Jones, Stuart Dwyer, Caitriona Row, Lucy Hine, and Kate Tolley.

To Peter Hubbard, Molly Gendell, Alison Hinchcliffe, Amelia Wood, Rachel Meyers and the whole brilliant team at Mariner Books.

To Marisa Vigilante and Tracy Behar at Little Brown, Spark for taking the book stateside.

To Mark Watson for making it all happen. To Jane Goldman for teaching me how to write long stuff. To Dan Swimer for the Knob-in-fan Persie joke (which got cut from this edition). To Justin Myers for his wisdom of words. To Gerry Farrell for the title. To Stephen McCrum for that first TV-writing job when I stumbled out of medicine. To Caroline Knight, my medical adviser ("Leave this bit out—it might actually stop people wanting children"). To Mark Davies for the odd bit of American "translation." To whoever makes Diplomático rum.

To so many former colleagues for jogging and sharing memories, especially Drs. Jones, Tanner, Gibson, Norbury, Trever, Henderson, van Hegan, Bonsall, Harvey, Heeps, Rehman, Bayliss, Saunders-hyphenvest, Laycock, McGinn, Lillie, Mansoori, Kupelian, Steingold, O'Neill, Biswas, Lieberman, Webster, Khan, Whitlock, and Moore.

And to Anna Welander, Megan McCluskie, Karl Webster, Zoe Waterman, Nikki Williams, Tim Bittlestone, Mike Wozniak, Jackson Sargeant, Cath Gagon, James Seabright, Paul Sullivan, Annie Cullum, Michael Howard, Trish Farrell, and everyone I've forgotten.

With no thanks whatsoever to Jeremy Hunt.

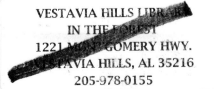